# Global Hair Care Secrets

# Table of Contents

# Preface

With this book, Mona strives to share her extensive knowledge and experience of hair care and treatments throughout nine countries. Explore the wonders of hair oils, mask recipes and ancient treatments to improve the quality of your hair, as well as their genetic, dietary and environmental impacts. Through practical guidance from an experienced expert, readers will find clear and simple advice for cultivating healthy, luscious locks. This book is an essential guide for anyone looking for a straightforward approach to nurturing their tresses. Mona holds an Australian hairdressing qualification and has an active presence on Instagram @mona_preen, here she shares tips, tricks and tutorials with her followers. The inspiration to write this book struck one day when she was washing a client's hair in a basin. She realised that the outcome of healthy hair without high porosity and damage is much more important than colour and hairstyle. So, Mona decided to search for countries with good hair history and write about their easy home remedies and oils to help people take better care of their hair.

# Introduction

Welcome to *Global Hair Care Secrets*! Written by Mona, a passionate hairdresser, this book shares her knowledge and experience with hair oils, recipes and treatments. From providing simple home-based mask recipes for improving one's hair quality to discovering some of the best hair globally, this book is an easy-to-follow guide for anyone seeking a comprehensive guide to hair care. Additionally, it provides insights into the key role genetics, diet and ancient hair treatments play in achieving healthy, luscious tresses.

Mona draws upon her experience to share tips and tricks for hair oil treatments gathered over many years. She highlights the importance of only oiling 1-2 times per week to maximise the benefit of oil nutrients and explains how over-oiling can attract dirt and strip the essential oils from the hair. Mona also emphasises the need for pregnant women or those with allergies to consult a physician before engaging in any hair remedies and treatments. Overall, this book provides an invaluable source of information to anyone interested in taking action towards attaining and maintaining perfect hair. With its clarity, simplicity and passion, Mona's book is the perfect guide to embarking on a healthy hair journey.

# Acknowledgements

I would like to express my sincere gratitude and appreciation to my husband, Dr Ali Aslani, for his tireless support and invaluable advice throughout the writing process. Your helpful tips have enabled me to achieve success, and I could not have done it without you. Thank you from the bottom of my heart. I am also grateful for the support of my beautiful girls , Kiana and Dayana .

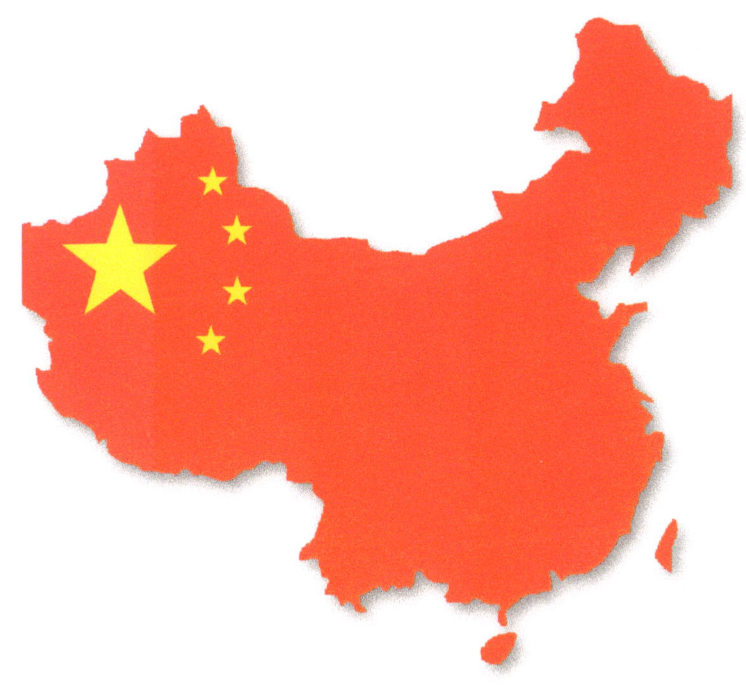

# China

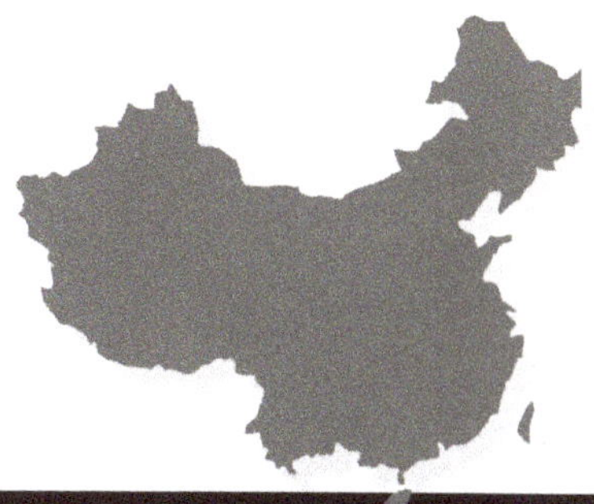

# Introduction

Chinese people have been blessed with dark, straight and silky hair that can instantly make anyone envious. Natural remedies and treatments are extremely popular in China, with traditional Chinese medicine, acupuncture, acupressure, etc., being all-natural methods to bring back health that have been successfully used for a very long time.

## Combing and massaging

Chinese people love combing and massaging their hair. They have special wood combs for this. These improve blood circulation on the scalp, thereby promoting hair growth. The history of massage is very old and it has been a part of traditional Chinese medicine forever. Regular massaging can help nourish the hair roots with oxygen and nutrients and is referred to as "qi" in China, meaning nourishing the body by the constant flow of energy. Spending every day and night combing and massaging for 3 minutes can help improve your hair drastically.

## Natural products

Chinese model Liu wen has shared haircare secrets from her hometown, Yongzhou. She says that she uses fruits of the Chinese soap-pod locust tree by boiling them in water and using the resulting mixture as shampoo. Chinese people also love fermented rice water,

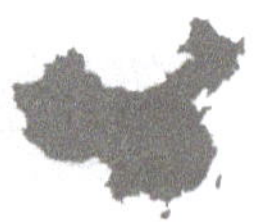

which is a protein-enriched rinse that will make your hair thicker and stronger. A detailed recipe for how to properly make fermented rice water is given below. Consuming ginseng, honeysuckles, seaweed and wheatgrass are all great for hair as well.

## Diet

It's no hidden secret that a healthy diet leads to good skin and hair, however, you might be unaware of some of the natural ingredients that are native to China that can help you stimulate hair growth. Liu wen also talks about her love for goji berries and Chinese red dates, saying she uses these in tea or congee to help achieve glowing skin. Both of these are packed with vitamins, minerals and antioxidants that are amazing for your hair, and not just your skin. Another model, Fei Fei Sun, describes how these two ingredients are present in everyone's diet in her hometown in China due to their health benefits.

## Avoid too much sun

Chinese beauty ideals include dark hair and pale skin, and therefore, they avoid the sun as much as possible and wear sunscreen. Sun is necessary for getting sufficient Vitamin D; however, too much exposure to UV radiation can lead to hair cuticle damage. The hair can appear brittle and discoloured, making it look rough and frizzy. Do not by any means avoid the sun completely, but protect your hair by wearing hats/scarves and sunscreen.

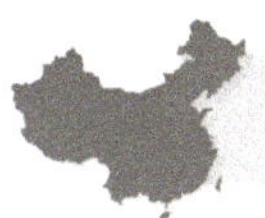



# Natural hair masks

## Fermented rice water rinse for hair growth

**Ingredients**

- 1 cup uncooked rice
- 4 cups water

The Red Yao women residing in the Huangluo town of China hold the Guinness World Record for "the world's longest hair village." These women have dark, strong, smooth and very long hair due to their traditional practice of soaking their hair in rice water. Rice water is rich in starch, amino acids, Vitamins B and E, and many minerals. It has inositol that will help to strengthen hair, reduce hair fall and stimulate hair growth. Amino acids help in smoothing and strengthening hair strands.

To make fermented rice water, rinse the rice properly and soak it in water for around 2 hours. Strain the liquid and let it ferment at room temperature for 3-4 days in a glass jar or earthenware pot, and cover it with a lid. You will know it's ready once it has a sour smell. You can ferment the rice water in the refrigerator as well for 3-4 weeks in a spray bottle. You can also add slices of ginger or oranges to it before fermenting for extra benefits.

For application, shampoo your hair first. Then mix 1 part rice water and 1 part normal water (around a cup each) and pour over your hair. Rinse after 10 minutes and repeat twice a week.

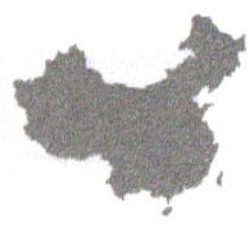

## Ginseng for hair growth

**Ingredients**

- 3-4 tbsp of coconut oil
- 1 capsule of Ginseng supplement

Ginseng has recently been gaining popularity for its numerous health benefits; however, it has been an important herb in East Asian countries for centuries. Several scientific studies have provided evidence for the remarkable properties of ginseng to boost hair growth. It can inhibit 5-alpha reductase and has many minerals, vitamins and antioxidants such as β-sitosterol and Linoleic acids that nourish the scalp. You can see its effects in terms of increased hair density and thickness and reduced inflammation.

Ginseng is rich in saponins called ginsenosides, which are the active molecules of ginseng helping in hair growth. A study in Korea suggested that ingestion of Red ginseng can be effective in enhancing hair density for patients with alopecia areata, which is an autoimmune disorder leading to hair loss in specific areas of the scalp. Applying ginseng on the scalp has also been proven scientifically to enhance hair growth.

Open up a capsule of ginseng supplement and coconut oil in a bowl. Mix it well and apply it to the scalp and massage gently for 5-10 minutes. Do this daily for the best results.

## Lemon-ginseng rinse for dandruff

**Ingredients**

- 2 tbsp lemon juice
- 4 tbsp ginseng OR 2 ginseng tea bags OR 2 ginseng capsules
- 2 cups water

Lemon has antimicrobial activity and does wonders for eliminating dandruff and itchiness. You'll see a notable difference after a single use! But do not go overboard with it as lemon can also be drying. Use it once or twice a week. Ginseng is rich in antioxidants and vitamins and has saponins, which are antibacterial and antifungal compounds that can help you get rid of that stubborn dandruff! It is effective against species of *Bacillus* that can cause dandruff.

Prepare ginseng tea by cutting fresh Ginseng roots and pouring hot water over them. Let it steep for a couple of minutes or until it's cooled down. You can also use instant Ginseng tea or ginseng supplements. Both are inexpensive and easy to find at a pharmacy or a health store. Add lemon juice and apply it with a squeeze or spray bottle. Keep it for an hour and rinse it with lukewarm water and a mild shampoo.

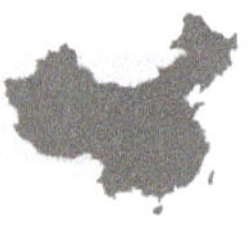

## Wheatgrass- A hair superfood

**Ingredients**

- ¼ cup fresh wheatgrass OR 2 tbsp wheatgrass powder

Wheatgrass corresponds to the young shoots of the wheat plant. These shoots are packed with nutrients that help in nourishing and detoxifying our bodies. Wheatgrass is a very rich source of chlorophyll, which is a strong antioxidant and detoxifying agent. Other than that, it is very high in Vitamins A, B, C, E and K and carotenoids. Minerals including iron, calcium, magnesium and sulfur are all also abundant. Seventeen different essential and non-essential amino acids make it an excellent source of nourishment for our hair. Including wheatgrass juice in our diet can help improve our hair health significantly. The topical application of wheatgrass juice also assists in increasing hair growth.

Wheatgrass can be used fresh or in dried powder form. For fresh wheatgrass, cut it and immediately either juice it in a blender or crush it with a mortar pestle and strain it. For powder, you can mix it in water to make a paste. Apply it to the scalp with a cotton ball and keep it for half an hour. Rinse it with a mild shampoo afterwards.

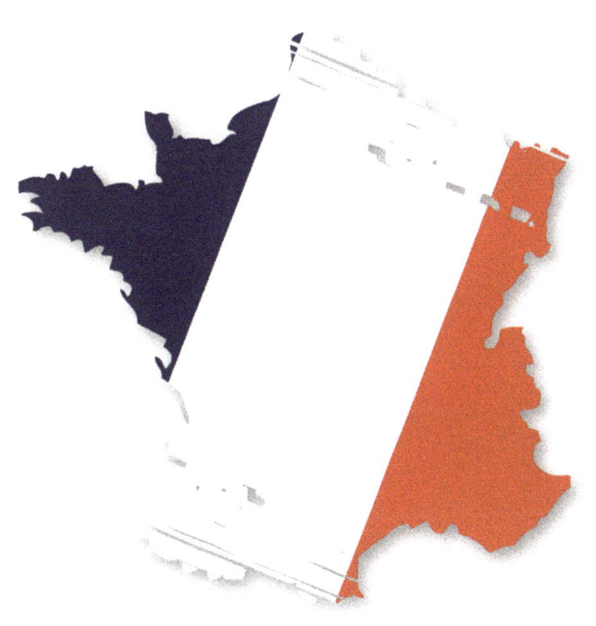

# FRANCE

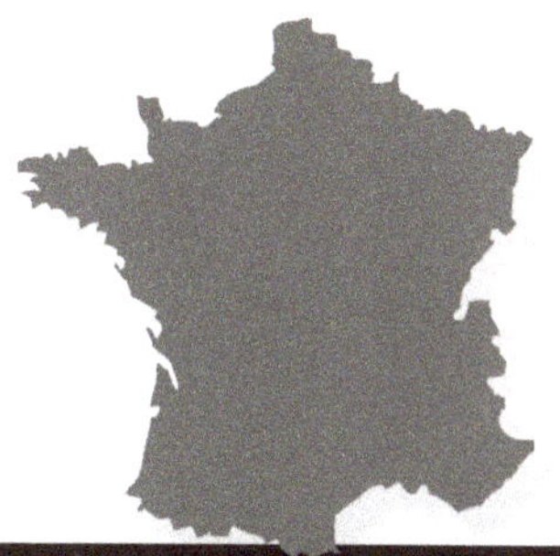

# Introduction

When we talk about France or French hair, the image that comes to our mind would probably be a soft and wavy, slightly dishevelled style that looks elegant yet effortless. This refers to the "French-girl hair" and is not at all difficult to achieve. Here are some secrets that can help you unlock your inner ingénue.

## Washing hair: Less is more

Washing your hair too often will strip the natural oils in your scalp. These oils are good for your hair and removing them leads to even more oil production as a feedback mechanism. Washing your hair twice a week can be a great routine but always adjust to your hair type and what suits you. A renowned French model, Caroline de Maigret, also recommends not washing your hair every day.

## Conditioner: Placement is important

French people always use a conditioner or a leave-in conditioner in their hair. However, only apply it to your ends and not the roots. Over conditioning can make the hair appear limp and unable to hold any shape or volume.

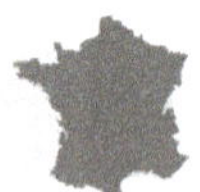

## The gentler, the better

People in France tend to avoid using harsh chemicals on their hair as they can damage it in the long run. They avoid products that are filled with silicones and sulfates and prefer formulations leaning toward the more natural and milder side. They also avoid harsh hair dyes that are filled with ammonia, peroxides and other nasty chemicals.

## Avoid heat

The French usually air dry their hair as this gives it more of a messy textured look and also prevents heat damage. If you want to prevent heat damage but cannot ditch the blow-dryer, make sure to use a heat protectant and use cooler settings.

## Don't brush your hair too much

Brushing is great for your hair as it improves blood circulation; however, over-brushing can be a real killjoy. Hair has a natural wave and volume that can be lost by brushing and it can make it appear frizzy. It can also lead to hair breakage. Instead, use a wide-toothed comb to prevent any hair ripping or breakage. France is famous for tortoiseshell combs and other accessories that are also exported to other countries.

## Volume is key

French people love bouncy voluminous hair and have their secrets to achieving that look. As they mostly have straight and silky hair, they use dry shampoo or texture spray (sea salt ones are a great option). A trick to achieve hair volume without any product is to sleep with slightly damp hair. Do not sleep with dripping wet hair though, as that can lead to follicle damage and hair breakage.

## Do not forget your weekly treatment

A very common practice in France is the use of weekly treatments. These treatments include hot oils, deep conditioners, hair masks, etc. A weekly treatment also allows them to spend less time on their hair during the weekdays. Although natural remedies are not something used by everyone in France all the time, they have their share of natural secrets. Some of the French hair masks that you can easily make at home are listed below.

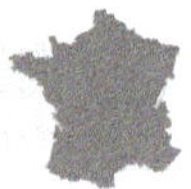

# Natural hair masks

## Clay and lavender oil hair mask for oily hair

**Ingredients**

- ¼ cup rhassoul clay
- 1 tbsp avocado oil
- 5 drops lavender essential oil
- 5 tbsp water or enough to make a paste

Rhassoul clay, also called red clay, is a reddish-brown clay and is a part of many skin and haircare formulations. It has detergent-like properties and therefore is used in shampoos. It is rich in magnesium and silicates due to the presence of stevensite as the major mineral. The clay will suck out any grease and impurities and will give the hair a natural shine. Clay has oil-absorbing properties and adding avocado oil will help you moisturize your hair. It will also strengthen hair in the long term.

Lavender oil is anti-bacterial, antifungal and anti-inflammatory. It has antioxidant properties and relieves skin conditions such as psoriasis and eczema. It contains phenols, tannins and flavonoids such as linalool, camphor, cineole, caffeic acid and triterpenes. These components of lavender oil help in improving blood circulation, have sudatory effects and provide a pleasant aroma that can have a calming/relaxing effect. It has also been reported to reduce hair loss and induce hair growth.

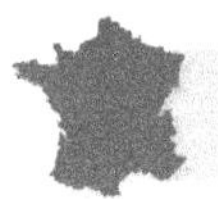



Mix clay and water to make a thick paste, add more or less water to adjust the consistency, and then add in the oils. Apply this only on your scalp and roots by sectioning your hair. Cover your hair so the clay does not dry out very fast. Leave it on for 30 minutes and rinse it off with warm water.

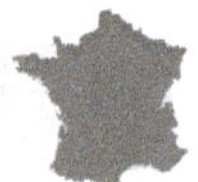

## Rosehip-peppermint hair oil for hair regrowth

**Ingredients**

- 2 tbsp jojoba oil
- 1 tsp rosehip oil
- 4 drops peppermint essential oil

Peppermint oil is native to Europe and has been part of French haircare for a long time. Studies have provided evidence that the topical application of peppermint oil stimulates hair follicles and helps in hair regrowth and improving hair density. Rosehip oil has an abundance of Vitamin C and A, plus omegas 3 and 6 fatty acids and is rich in antioxidants such as lycopene and tocopherols. It is also a great source of squalene and collagen. Jojoba oil also has a significant amount of tocopherols and is a rich source of Vitamins A and D.

Mix the oils, massage them on your scalp gently, and leave it for 1 hour. Rinse it off with shampoo after. Both jojoba and rosehip oil are very moisturizing and peppermint has a high regrowth potential. Regular use of this oil can help anyone who's looking to fill thinning spots and enhance overall hair density.

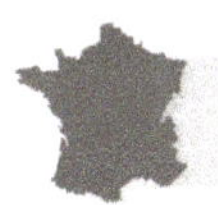



## Avocado-egg protein mask

**Ingredients**

- 2 avocados
- 2 eggs
- 2 tbsp olive oil
- 1 tsp raw honey

Many of us have dreamt of long healthy and shiny locks, but growing your hair can be a challenge especially if it is weak and brittle. Hair is made up of proteins and requires those building blocks to keep its elasticity, shine and strength. Adding a protein mask to your haircare routine will ensure faster hair growth and less chopping due to damage. Eggs and avocados are great sources of protein, omega-3 fatty acids and various vitamins and minerals. Honey is a natural humectant and provides moisture and shine to hair.

Blend everything and add it to a squeeze bottle or a bowl. If the mixture is too thick, you can add more olive oil. Apply the mixture from the roots to the ends and completely saturate your hair. Cover your hair and let the mask do its magic for 30 minutes. Rinse and condition afterwards. Use this once a week or fortnight.

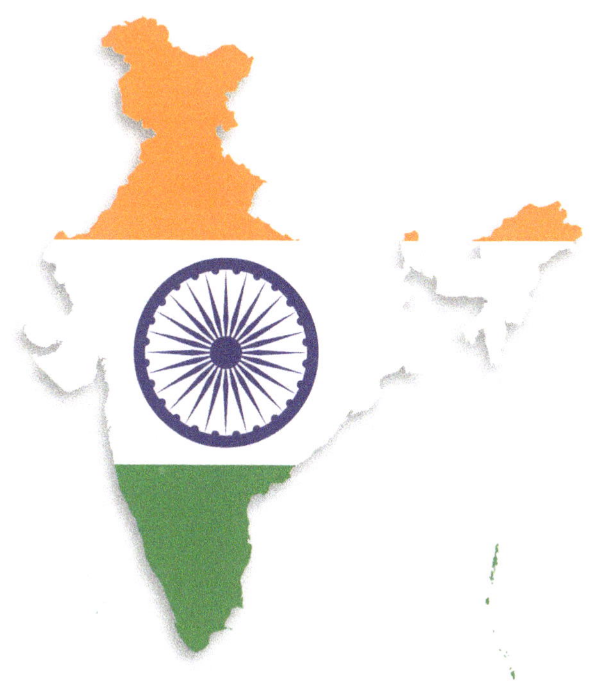

# India

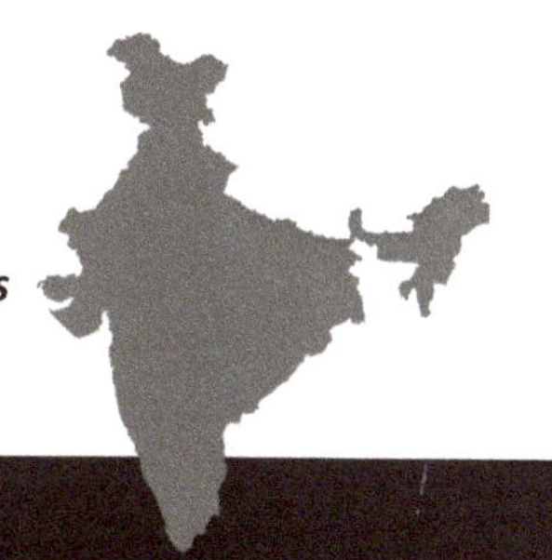

# Introduction

If you know something about Indian culture or have heard ancient Indian stories, you will have noticed that all the queens or ladies are portrayed with long, beautiful, heavy and shiny hair down to their knees. Likewise, the princes, kings and saints are described as having thick and luscious hair on their shoulders with long thick beards. The old paintings of Indian queens, kings and all those other characters worth remembering say it all: heavenly, beautiful hair.

Even if we talk about the present time, Indians still have this quality of divinely beautiful, thick, long and luscious hair. Almost all the older ladies in India, despite their old ages, have blacker, shinier and denser hair compared to other regions. Of course, the new haircare products didn't even use to be available in some areas of India, but still, Indians somehow managed to slay with their healthy, dreamy and Rapunzel-like hair.
The secret behind Indian hair

## The question here arises:

- Do Indians know some witchcraft that makes their hair grow like magic?
- Is this due to some old divine blessing?
- Is it simply genetic for Indians to have such beautiful hair?

And many more questions. But, the truthful answer is science.

Whether we're talking about Indian haircare secrets or the secrets behind any other magical trick, there's always science behind

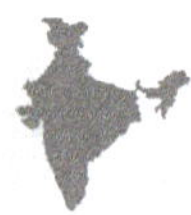

them. Sometimes chemical science, space science, biological science and sometimes..."AYURVEDA SCIENCE."

Ayurveda science is used for Indian haircare and skin care, healing and medication. But, here we'll shed light on haircare secrets. Various Indian haircare secrets are deeply embedded in Indian culture, where Ayurveda science plays a significant role.

## AYURVEDA SCIENCE

The word Ayurveda translates to "Ayuhr" as life and "Veda" as science. So that means "Science of Life." It uses nature as healing, and it's the oldest medical system of survival in the world. This science uses the goodness and quality of nature in herbal medications, specialized diets, meditation, yoga, acupressure and massage, etc. There's no doubt that—more than any advanced chemical formulation—these herbs and Ayurvedic techniques have done wonders for hair growth. So, let's see how it works for hair growth.

## Ayurveda- The witchcraft for Indian hair

The best part about this traditional Ayurvedic Indian haircare is that the methods are entirely natural and have no side effects. Most importantly, the ancient Ayurvedic Indian hair growth secrets are very effective. Ayurveda relies on 3 basic elements:

## MASSAGING

This is a very basic idea: Your hair will grow better if your scalp is healthier. Applying blends of specific herbs and natural oils rich in proteins, vitamins and other vitally essential minerals to the scalp in desirable amounts and massaging sometimes makes blood circulation better. This further nourishes the roots of your hair to make them grow faster and healthier.

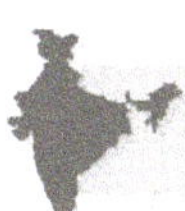



## DIET

Diet also plays a vital role in hair health. If your body doesn't have the right amount of nutrients, vitamins and minerals, it won't be able to process hair growth, and thus you'll lose hair. That's why a proper diet is vital for hair growth. Proteins, zinc, iron, Vitamins A, B, B12 C, D and E, and folate and selenium-enriched foods must be included in our diet to boost hair growth.

## ACUPRESSURES

This is a technique in which pressure is applied to the acupoints on the body's meridians. Thus, it stimulates circulation and heals the body from the inside, triggering hair's growth process. This technique involves stretching, acupressure massage and some other methods.

Now, let's talk about some other traditions:

## OILING

Oiling is one of the best ancient Indian hair growth secrets; it's the crucial one to get the desired hair growth. According to the ancient Indian practice of Ayurveda, washing and oiling your hair once a week is recommended. If your hair is exceptionally dry or has a lot of dandruff, it's recommended to oil your hair twice or thrice a week, but not more than thrice.

The oils mentioned are coconut oil, olive oil, castor oil, almond oil, jojoba oil, etc. The term "Indian hair oiling rituals" refers to the application of these oils on the scalp for extended durations. Massaging oil on the scalp leads to proper absorption of qualities of oil leading to shiny and long hair. Pollutants, heat, chemicals and ultraviolet radiation damage hair, but oiling deeply moisturizes and conditions from the roots and boosts a scalp's health.

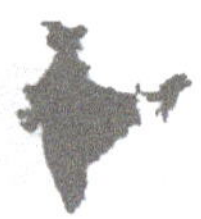

Renowned Indian actress and former Miss World, **Aishwarya Rai Bachchan**, has also shared her love for oiling. When asked about her secret for getting such healthy and beautiful hair, she talks about essential oils, a healthy diet and an adequate amount of hydration as crucial components that should not be ignored. She loves to apply homemade and herbal hair masks and prefers them over commercially available ones. Her favourite hair mask is an avocado and yoghurt hair mask.

## How it works

Oiling helps in maintaining the natural oils of the hair. It stimulates the hair follicle for amazing hair growth and improves the flow of blood, enhancing scalp health. It also exfoliates the hair follicles that may be clogged by dead skin and flakes. This traditional Indian haircare method works in almost all cases.

One should, however, be careful about oiling hair too much as it might lead to other issues. Balance here is the key!

## The right way to oil your hair

- Lightly heat some oil in a bowl.
- Using your fingers, gently apply the oil to your scalp.
- Massage in a light circular motion with fingertips, initiating from the middle of your head, leading outward.
- After massaging for 5-10 minutes, apply oil down the lengths of your hair.
- Comb and secure your hair in a loose braid.
- You'll get the best results if you do this before going to bed, as the oil will work overnight to nourish your scalp. Or you can do this 6-7 hours before you shower.
- Use mild shampoo to wash your hair. Try not to over- or under-wash.

Here are some of the proven ancient Indian herbal oils that can be used to promote your hair growth as well as scalp health. These herbal oils are a powerhouse of various types of vitamins, proteins and minerals.

I recommend you go through the descriptions of these hair oils and decide on the ones you could use for yourself. You can also go for a composite plan of using these oils on alternate days.

## COCONUT OIL

Coconut oil is one of the most popular oils; it is often said to be the best oil to use on your hair to reduce protein loss and keep it looking healthy. Being enriched with lauric acid, it has a long and straight structure that gets easily absorbed into the hair shaft.

When applied to the hair before washing, coconut oil has been shown to reduce protein loss more effectively than mineral oils. Your hair is most vulnerable to damage when it's wet. Applying oil to your hair before and after you wash it helps protect it from damage.

### Other benefits of coconut oil for hair

- ❖ Lice prevention
- ❖ Sun protection
- ❖ Dandruff treatment
- ❖ Hair loss prevention.

### Different ways that you can use coconut oil for hair

- ❖ As a conditioner

Shampoo your hair as usual and then comb coconut oil through your hair, from the midsection to the ends.

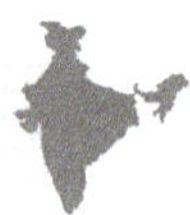

- As a hair mask

Rub coconut oil through your hair and let it sit for a few hours (or even overnight) before washing it out.

- As a scalp treatment

Massage a small amount of coconut oil into your scalp before bed. Leave it overnight and wash it off with shampoo in the morning.

**Caution: It's recommended not to use coconut oil in excess.**

## Other oils

### AMLA OIL

This is an ancient herb that is made using a herbal plant, the Indian gooseberry. While all parts of the amla tree are believed to hold medicinal benefits, amla fruits are very high in Vitamin C and several other antioxidants and nutrients.

### CASTOR OIL

Castor oil is a nutrient-rich vegetable oil extracted from castor beans. In its primary element, the oil is clear or has a yellow colour. You can also make black castor oil produced by roasting or boiling the beans.

This miracle oil hydrates and moisturizes a dry scalp and provides additional shine to the hair. Castor oil is suitable for all hair types, including frizzy hair. You can even use it to thicken your eyebrows and obtain denser and longer eyelashes.

### ALMOND OIL

Using almond oil on your hair gives it a softer texture over time. Almond oil can make hair more robust and less prone to split ends, which means your hair growth won't be slowed by losing hair that becomes damaged. In addition, almond oil contains high amounts of Vitamin E, a natural and trusted source of antioxidants. When antioxidants combat the environmental stress around your hair, your hair looks younger and healthier. Almond oil can also be used to treat flaky scalp (seborrheic dermatitis) and scalp psoriasis. Almond oil has been used to treat dry scalp conditions in Ayurvedic medicine.

## BRAIDING

Braiding is one of the most common and frequently used hairstyles in India. However, many of us are not aware that it's not just a hairstyle, but also a proven way to get healthier hair growth.

Keeping your hair in braids reduces friction between your hair and pillow, reducing hair breakage.

### How it works

Apart from giving your hair a natural wavy texture, it also keeps your hair detangled and thus prevents breakage and promotes growth.

## BALAYAM TECHNIQUE

This technique was invented by ancient Indian Rishi Munis about 5,000 years ago.

Balayam means hair exercise. This combination of yoga and acupressure is an easy and effective option to prevent premature hair whitening and loss, which you also can find in yoga.

Balayam is a straightforward yoga technique that helps in hair regrowth. The method works for many people, though it does not work for some people. It depends on people's DNA structure, body nature and immune system.

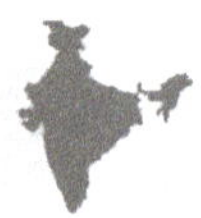

If you are very upset with your hair loss and are going toward baldness ahead of time, one of the solutions to this problem can be Balayam.

## How it works

Rubbing nails together increases hair growth. This is because the nerve endings in our fingertips are linked to the scalp. So, when you rub your nails together, the friction you create affects nerves in the scalp. This, in turn, increases blood flow and stimulates hair growth.

To get the expected results, do nail rubbing exercises daily for an hour or in 4 sessions of 15 minutes each. The anticipated results will occur only after a long regular practice of at least 6-7 months.

## The right way to do Balayam

When you rub your nails, after 5 minutes, you may feel tingling in your nails. This means you are doing it correctly.

When you rub them, your scalp will get hot.

In the first 1-2 months, hair fall increases because the stem cells work. This is the third way of identifying if you are doing Balayam the right way.

## Best time to practice this technique

Early morning and evening is the ideal Balayam yoga time, but try to practice it on an empty stomach.

# Natural hair masks

## Hibiscus hair mask

**Ingredients**

- 3 to 4 Hibiscus leaves
- 1 Hibiscus flower (red ones are the best)
- 3-4 tbsp lukewarm water
- 2-3 tbsp coconut oil
- 1 non-plastic bowl

This hair mask works to enhance and protect the natural colour of your hair by preventing premature greying. It also protects hair from damage. Make a solution for weak roots as hibiscus is known to strengthen them.

**Best for DRY HAIR**

1. Wash hibiscus petals with water to remove any dirt and soil, then soak the leaves and flowers in water for 10 minutes. Next, simply crush and mash the flowers using your hands.
2. The liquid will start to bubble up and deepen; when it becomes slimy, it's time to use it. Simply strain it using a strainer. You will get an oily liquid that mostly is yellowish or golden in colour.
3. Now you can add your coconut oil to this liquid. Keep in mind you can simply use this blend even without coconut oil.
4. You can apply this pack to your hair before taking shower or at any time.

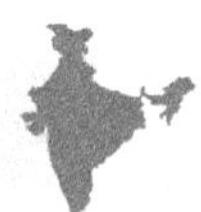

5. Keep the hair mask on for 5-10 minutes and then rinse it with water. You will definitely feel its cooling and refreshing effect.
6. It not only nourishes the roots but makes the hair smooth and silky as well!

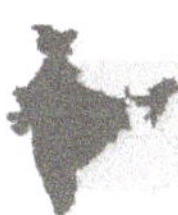



## Amla-curd hair mask

**Ingredients**

- 2 tbsp amla powder
- 1 tbsp shikakai powder
- 1 bowl smoothened yoghurt
- 1 tbsp lemon juice

The curd will make your scalp healthier and nourished, and it will prevent dandruff. Shikakai and amla together will work as natural conditioners for your hair, resulting in spa-like silky-smooth and luscious hair.

**Best for DANDRUFF PRONE SCALP**

1. Take the required amount of amla and shikakai powder.
2. Mix using warm water and make a thick paste. Leave it to set overnight.
3. The following morning, add yoghurt and again make a smooth paste.
4. Let it stand for at least an hour. After an hour, add lemon juice and mix.
5. Apply on your scalp and follow down the length. Make a bun and leave the mask.
6. Wash hair after 1 hour and enjoy the results from the very first use.

Your hair will become silkier and softer, like it is after being conditioned.

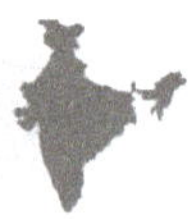

## Stale and sour curd mask

**Ingredients**

- 1 old rotten banana
- 4-5 tbsp stale and sour curd
- 2 tbsp aloe vera gel
- 1 egg
- 3-4 tbsp lemon juice

This is the ultimate haircare mask for almost all types of hair. Specifically, it treats hair loss problems. But also, you can enjoy smooth, softer and luscious hair after each use. Further, it will make your scalp nourished and healthier. You can also call this hair mask a multi-ingredient hair mask.

**Best for: HAIR LOSS**

1. Take the aloe plant and wash it. Let the yellow part wash away. Soak it in water for a few minutes and extract the white, clean gel part.
2. Put that into a bowl, then add egg, sour curd and the rotten banana.
3. Mix the ingredients well. Make sure there are no lumps left. (You can use a mixer for a better paste)
4. Apply to the scalp as well as hair length.
5. Leave for 30 minutes. Now, use that lemon juice and mix it with 1 glass of water. Set it aside.
6. Wash with normal water. Now, wash your hair with lemon juice to remove the smell of eggs.

Enjoy your beautiful hair!

The best part about this recipe is that it uses waste and old food ingredients and works so effectively.

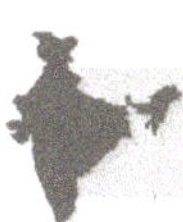



## Here's the scientific secret that many aren't aware of!

Sour curd is enriched with Vitamin B5 and Vitamin D. It's also loaded with essential amino acids, zinc, potassium and magnesium. Rubbing it on the scalp and applying it throughout the length will feed your scalp and hair with all the essential nutrition, resulting in smooth, shiny hair and a healthier scalp.

## How to prepare sour curd at home

- Boil milk and leave it in a container to cool down.
- Add half a tbsp curd or lemon juice. Mix it well.
- Keep the container in a warm place.
- Refrigerate after the milk gets frozen and thickened up.
- Now, this is the fresh curd that is used in food.
- For sour curd, you need to let it stale up and older to get ready to be used on hair. Placing it in a warmer place or outside the refrigerator can speed up the process. Once the curd gets soured up, you can smell the sourness. Now you can use it to prepare a hair mask.

People often use fresh curd, but sour curd shows better results as it has more nutritious elements for hair health.

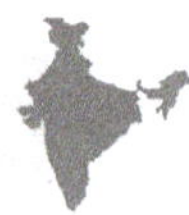

## Rotten banana mask

**Ingredients**

- 2 old rotten bananas
- 2 tbsp aloe vera gel
- 1 egg
- 3-4 tbsp lemon juice

This is the ultimate haircare mask for almost all types of hair. Particularly, it treats hair loss problems. Regardless, you can enjoy smooth, softer and luscious hair after each use. Also, it will make your scalp nourished and healthier. You can also call this hair mask a multi-ingredient hair mask.

**Best for: HAIR LOSS**

1. Take the aloe plant and wash it. Let the yellow part wash away. Soak it in water for a few minutes and extract the white, clean gel part.
2. Put the gel into a bowl. Add the egg and the rotten banana.
3. Mix the ingredients well. Make sure there are no lumps left. (You can use a mixer for a better paste)
4. Apply on the scalp as well as hair length.
5. Leave for 30 minutes. Now, use the lemon juice and mix it with 1 glass of water. Keep it aside.
6. Wash with normal water. Now, wash your hair with lemon juice to remove the smell of eggs.

Enjoy beautiful hair!

The best part about this recipe is that it uses waste and old food ingredients and works so effectively.

## Neem and yoghurt mask for dandruff

**Ingredients**

- ½ cup yoghurt
- A handful of neem leaves OR 1 tbsp neem powder OR 10 drops neem essential oil
- 3 cloves of garlic
- 1 tbsp onion oil

Neem is a very powerful antimicrobial agent and has been proven effective against dandruff-causing fungi. Yoghurt is rich in protein and Vitamin B5, so it will moisturize and condition your hair. Probiotics in yoghurt can also help in controlling dandruff due to their anti-fungal action.

Allicin, the main active compound in garlic, corresponds to its anti-fungal and anti-bacterial properties. Many studies have reported the efficacy of garlic and onions against various dandruff-causing fungi. Both of them have organosulfur compounds, which causes them to be pungent. These compounds are antioxidants and prevent free radical damage to the skin. All these ingredients are anti-inflammatory as well and will soothe an itchy and irritated scalp.

Blend everything in a blender to make a thick mask. Apply it to your scalp and roots and cover it with a shower cap or plastic bag. Leave it on for an hour at least and rinse it thoroughly with shampoo.

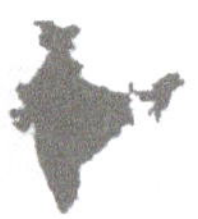

## Mustard and amla oil for grey hair

**Ingredients**

- 1 cup mustard oil
- 2 tbsp henna powder
- ½ tbsp fenugreek powder
- ½ tbsp amla (Indian gooseberry) powder

Amla has been used in India for centuries as a fruit and as an ayurvedic remedy. It is a highly rich source of Vitamin C, richer even than oranges and lemons! Also, it's a great source of amino acids, minerals, flavonoids and tannins. Indians use amla for their hair to prevent and reverse greying of hair. Although no evidence is available to back up this claim, research has proven amla to be effective in promoting hair growth due to its 5-alpha reductase inhibitory properties. Henna has been used in India as a natural dye forever and is a great natural alternative to chemicals. Fenugreek seeds are rich in lecithin, which is a natural emollient. It is also rich in amino acids, vitamins, fatty acids and saponins, all of which provide nourishment to the hair. It will also prevent dandruff due to its anti-inflammatory and anti-microbial properties.

Heat an iron utensil, and at a very low flame, cook the oil for 5 minutes. Iron utensils leach iron into the oil, which the hair will benefit from. Stir is constantly in between. The oil will turn a dark, almost black colour. Switch off the gas, cover the iron utensil with the oil and let it sit for 24 hours. The oil will thicken and will be very dark in colour. Strain the oil and store it in a glass jar. The shelf life of this will be 2 months. For effective results, use this oil 3-4 times a week on your scalp, roots and ends. For application, apply this oil overnight and shampoo the next day. This oil will turn your already grey hair black, and the new hair growth will be dark as well.

## Herbal hair oil for hair growth

### Ingredients

- 2 cups coconut oil
- 3-4 sprigs of curry leaves
- 1 small onion (chopped)
- 4 hibiscus flowers (Red preferred)
- 10 hibiscus leaves
- 2 tbsp nigella seeds (black seeds)
- 2 tbsp fenugreek seeds

Ayurvedic herbal oils are a staple of every Indian home. These oils, as the name indicates, are infused with various herbs. Countless varieties of these oils exist and every household might have a version of its own. This herbal oil is enriched with ingredients that will promote hair growth and will make your hair softer and stronger over time. Coconut oil is one of the most common oils used in India for hair care. It is rich in a short-chain fatty acid called lauric acid, which is linear and small in size and, therefore, can penetrate the hair shaft easily. Curry leaves are rich in amino acids, beta carotene (Vitamin A) and Vitamin B, such as nicotinic acid, Vitamin C and important minerals required for hair growth such as calcium, phosphorus, Iron, zinc and copper. Plus, it is a powerful natural antioxidant.

According to traditional Indian texts, hibiscus can be used to promote hair growth and prevent greying of hair. A scientific study has shown that both the leaves and flowers of hibiscus are effective in promoting hair growth. Nigella seeds are rich in omega 3 and omega 6 fatty acids and various amino acids. It helps in improving blood circulation and promoting hair growth on the scalp.

For this oil, prepare a double boiler by placing a utensil on top of simmering water. Melt the coconut oil, and add each ingredient to

it. Let this mixture heat and infuse for an hour on a very low flame. After that, let the oil rest at room temperature for another hour. Strain the oil and store it in a glass jar. Apply this oil for 2 hours or overnight and use it twice a week.

In an Interview with *Vogue*, Famous Bollywood and Hollywood actress **Priyanka Chopra** shared the secret behind her thick, silky and luscious hair. The ingredients she mentioned for the mask were full-fat yoghurt, 1 tsp honey and 1 egg. She said to leave it on for 30 minutes and rinse it off with lukewarm water.

## Other ingredients for hair

### Henna

Another ancient Indian hair growth secret that has been a part of the Indian haircare routine for centuries, Henna, was very effective for hair growth.

It's multifunctional as it has been used to colour hair, have gorgeous mehndi and even repel insects.

Henna can be used with mustard oil to prevent hair fall.

### How it works

As an ingredient for Indian haircare, it makes hair stronger and shinier and reduces hair fall. Being enriched with antifungal and antibacterial properties, it helps in protecting the scalp from various infections.

### Shikakai

Amongst the most famous ancient Indian hair growth secrets, this traditional Indian haircare method is also very effective.

Shikakai, also called 'Fruit for hair,' is a natural herbal product used to cleanse and protect the hair. It can be used to make homemade shampoos that are chemical-free. Its benefits range from strengthening hair to fighting dandruff, delaying grey hair, preventing lice from detangling your hair and making it shine.

## How it works

Shikakai naturally strengthens the hair and promotes hair growth. In addition, its antifungal properties provide nutrition to the scalp and help to cure dandruff.

It fights infections and maintains a healthy pH level of the scalp.

It's indeed one of the best options to promote natural hair growth. Also, it helps in preventing premature greying of hair.

## Traditional TIP

- Make a schedule for your haircare.
- There are lots of theories about hair, beauty and skin routines.
- One theory is how the moon calendar may influence what days you should focus on your beauty and wellness.
- According to this theory, the best time for haircare is the days when the moon is in Leo and Virgo.
- That means you have a window of about 4 days each month to get your hair done. You might find this ridiculous, but it does not cost a penny, so it is worth trying.

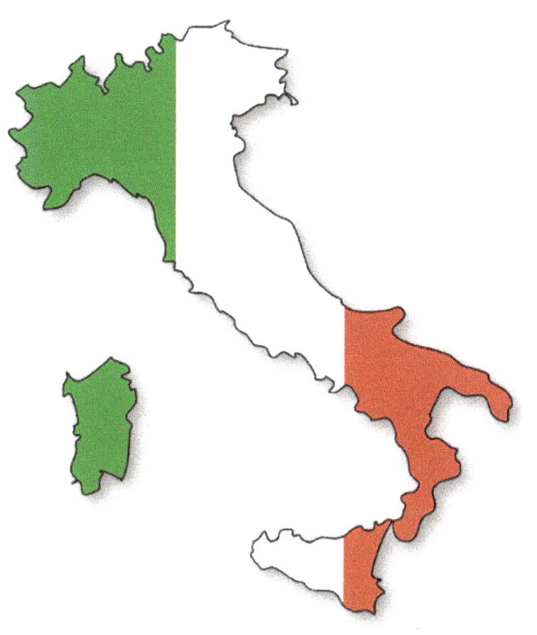

# Italy

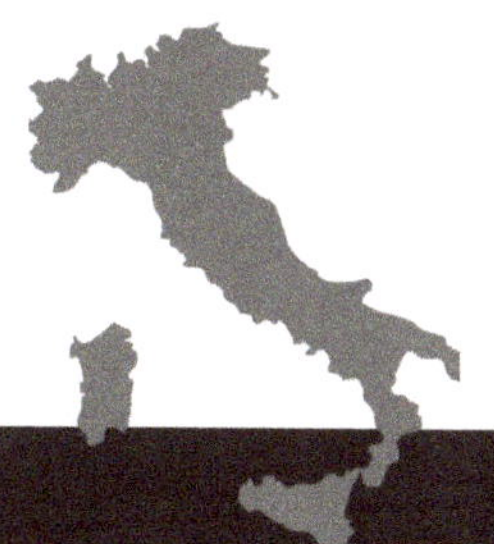

# Introduction

When walking down the streets of Milan, you will be greeted by beautiful radiant women with luscious manes that are full of volume and bounce. Italy, the land of pizza and pasta, the best creation to ever exist, is also home to many beauties such as Monica Bellucci and Missoni Clan. Putting effort into becoming your best not only involves your looks but also feeling your best. The Italians put great emphasis on healthy lifestyle choices and a stress-free environment and that reflects in their appearance as well.

## Olive oil -Italian holy grail

It is no hidden fact that the Italians love their olive oil and they put it in literally everything. With food, on the skin, to hair—there is not a single place where olive is deemed futile. The Italian grandmas have been using olive oil on their hair to nourish and moisturize for centuries and are passing this trend down to the next generations. A famous Italian actress and model, Sophia Loren, has shared that her secret is rubbing olive oil in her hair. Use a little bit of extra virgin oil every night on your ends to have soft and manageable hair throughout the day. Some hot treatments are also mentioned below in the recipes section.

## Italians love the sun (wear sunscreen though)

Sun usually gets unnecessary hate due to the rise of skin cancers. But sunlight is an extremely important natural source of Vitamin D. Vitamin D is amazing for hair health; it strengthens the hair and makes it appear radiant and healthy. Its deficiency can lead to severe hair loss. Italians love the sun and don't shy away from a good tan. Just use a hat, and tons of sunscreen, and avoid tanning beds at all costs! And you will be golden.

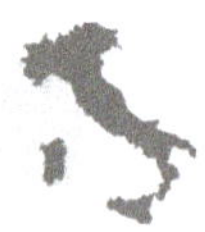

## Love for quality and authenticity

Italy is a country of refined taste, with simple dishes but quality ingredients. Having a good natural product is a very important tool for maintaining good health. Common ingredients used such as olive oil, basil, rosemary, etc., are all strong antioxidants and help fight against free radical damage. Unless you are getting proper nutrients, no hair remedy can provide you with the desired benefits. When asked about her hair secrets, Gilda Ambrosio, an Italian influencer, says that she always drinks 1 healthy juice per day.

## Go natural

Italians love to wear their hair in natural colours and do not use a lot of heat to protect their hair. There is nothing wrong with bleaching hair, but continuous bleaching can damage the hair to the point of no return. Consider getting highlights as these can give you a similar beautiful look but reduces the level of potential damage.

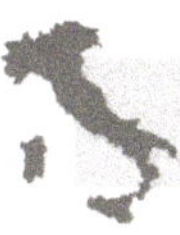



# Natural hair masks

## Stinging nettle-infused oil for dandruff and hair fall

**Ingredients**

- 1-part dried nettle leaves
- 3-parts grapeseed oil

Stinging nettle, although a weed, has great therapeutic importance and has been used for treating various diseases for centuries. It is rich in flavonoids that correspond to its anti-inflammatory and antioxidant properties. It is high in essential amino acids and various vitamins and minerals. Studies have reported evidence of nettle leaves and roots as inhibitors of 5-alpha reductase, which produces DHT, the main culprit of male and female pattern baldness. Its antimicrobial and anti-inflammatory properties are great for combating dandruff.

Chop the nettle leaves finely, and put them in an airtight, dark glass jar. Fill the jar with oil, cover it and let it infuse at room temperature for 4-6 weeks. You can also try the quick method, i.e., simmer the oil-nettle mixture on top of a double boiler for 5 hours, making sure that the water is not boiling but only simmering. After infusion, strain the oil and it is good to go. Apply this oil once a week to get rid of dandruff and for reducing hair fall.

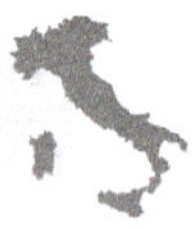

## Rosemary-sage hair tonic for oily hair

**Ingredients**

- ¼ cup fresh rosemary leaves
- 4-5 sage leaves
- ¼ cup fresh aloe vera
- 1 tbsp coconut oil

Rosemary is excellent for reducing hair fall and inducing hair regrowth. A study showed that it's as effective as 2% Minoxidil for regrowing hair. It stimulates the scalp, enhances blood circulation and helps in eliminating dandruff. Aloe vera provides hydration to the hair without making the hair oily or limp. This mask will control hair fall, excess sebum and dandruff and will improve the overall quality of your hair.

Blend everything and strain it with a cheesecloth. Apply this paste to the scalp and roots, and leave it for an hour. Rinse with a mild shampoo.

You can also mix this mask with any deep conditioner of your choice; it'll help to strengthen the hair that way as well.

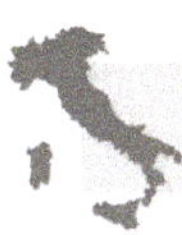



## Rosemary oil for alopecia and hair growth

**Ingredients**

- 10 drops rosemary essential oil
- 1 tbsp olive oil
- 1 tbsp almond oil

Alopecia is one of the prevalent hair issues today both in men and women. Although not harmful physically, it can severely affect a person mentally and lower their self-esteem and confidence. Androgenic alopecia is one of the major types of alopecia. It is commonly referred to as male or female pattern baldness. As the name indicates, it is caused by an excess of androgens, i.e., testosterone converted to Dihydrotestosterone by an enzyme called 5-alpha reductases in the hair follicles. Rosemary leaf extract is shown to inhibit 5-alpha reductase and promote hair regrowth in mice. In clinical trials, rosemary has proven to be as effective as minoxidil for inducing new hair growth.

Mix rosemary, olive oil and almond oil together. Warming up the oil before applying it helps to stimulate blood circulation and better absorption. You can use different carrier oils as well. Apply this oil for 2 hours and rinse it off with a shampoo.

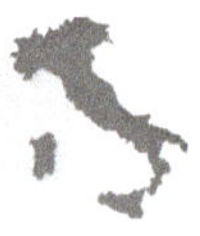

## Chamomile tea rinse for hair growth and lightening

**Ingredients**

- 1 tbsp chamomile tea OR 2 tea bags
- 1 cup water

We have all heard about the relaxing and de-stressing properties of drinking chamomile tea. However, the benefits of this plant go well beyond that. Topical use of chamomile tea promotes healthier, shinier hair. Anti-inflammatory compounds can alleviate an itchy, dry scalp that can lead to dandruff. It has been traditionally used as a hair lightener and has been part of different hair dye formulations. This hair-lightening property is due to the presence of a flavonoid called apigenin. Recent studies have found that apigenin also aids in hair growth. This rinse will lighten your hair without causing any damage. On the contrary, this will help you repair it.

Steep the tea for 5 minutes in hot water and let it cool. Pour it over your hair and make sure your hair is properly coated with it. Leave this mixture on the hair for 30 minutes. You can also use a spray bottle for a less messy application. Do this after shampooing and then rinse with water.

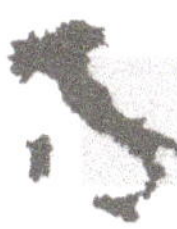



## Chamomile hair oil for hair growth and lightening

**Ingredients**

- 10 drops chamomile essential oil
- 3-4 tbsp jojoba or any carrier oil

We are all familiar with the possible damages caused by using bleach on our hair. Although tempting, lightening hair with chemicals can leave our hair dry, frizzy and in severe cases, broken. If you do not have access to chamomile tea but need something for a dry scalp type, then do not worry. Chamomile essential oil is equally efficacious and will improve the quality of your hair significantly. Chamomile essential oil has soothing benefits and is reported to relieve migraines as well. It is also reported to have anti-inflammatory and antimicrobial activity and is rich in antioxidants.

Mix the oils and apply the mixture to your scalp and hair length. Gently massage your hair to improve blood circulation on your scalp. Wait at least an hour before washing it off.

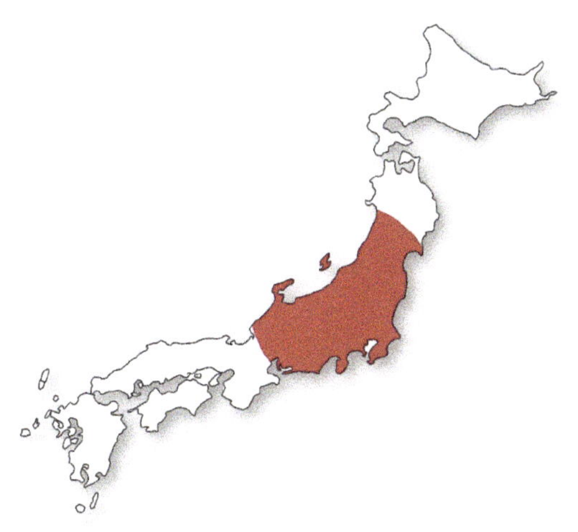

# JAPAN

# Introduction

Japanese women are known for having beautiful and radiant skin and hair. There is an old Japanese saying that translates to "beautiful hair can make any woman beautiful." If you think about Japanese women, a picture of someone with pale skin and very dark, silky hair comes to mind. Japanese hair ideals are for it to be black, silky and straight. For hundreds if not thousands of years, Japan has been using its natural remedies to achieve and maintain those ideals.

Let's dive into some of Japan's ancient secrets that have helped them to achieve their beautiful and luscious locks!

## The Japanese obsession with scalp care and spas:

If you have ever visited Japan, you will be familiar with their hair spas dedicated to scalp care. These are very popular in Japan and claim to cleanse, detox and rejuvenate the scalp by deep cleansing and massaging. These treatments help in improving blood circulation and unclogging pores. The scalp is often neglected and these treatments provide much-needed attention and care. You can make your scrub by mixing olive oil with Adzuki powder and gently massaging it on the scalp. Adzuki or red bean powder is non-abrasive and will therefore gently exfoliate.

## Wooden combs (Tsuge) in Japan:

In Japan, people prefer to comb multiple times a day and have special combs for that purpose. Tsuge is a boxwood tree used for creating these combs. This wood is not easy to find and each comb is handcrafted; therefore, these combs can be expensive. However, the durability of this comb makes it a good investment. The wood has natural oils that prevent the hair from tugging on it and breaking.

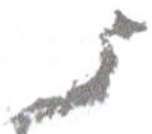

These combs assist in stimulating blood flow to the scalp and also distribute the natural oils across the hair evenly. People also soak their combs in camellia oil once every 3 months for the added benefits of a smooth and slick comb.

## Camellia oil: The holy grail of Japan

This is the most widely used and loved oil in Japan and is also a component of many hair and skincare products. Camellia oil, also called tea seed oil, is the cold-pressed oil extracted from the flowering species of *Camellia japonica* (Tsubaki) and referred to as Tsubaki oil in Japan. The flowers for this oil are red or pink called yabu, and therefore, the oil is called yabu-tsubaki oil. The oil is lightweight and golden in colour, and is most popular as a leave-in oil for softer and more manageable hair. It is high in good fatty acids, vitamins and minerals. It contains twice as much Vitamin E as olive oil and also contains more monounsaturated fatty acids (almost 90%). It is also abundant in squalene and flavonoids. The highest form of fatty acids in this oil is omegas 6 and 9, which will penetrate the hair shaft and provide moisture and softness to the hair.

The best or most common method for the application of this oil is after a shower, with a few drops on slightly damp hair to lock in moisture. You can also apply this before shampoo as an oil treatment on the scalp and ends.

A Japanese kimono expert, Junko Sophie Kakizaki, has also mentioned using camellia oil on her scalp before washing her hair. Along with that, she also mentioned sakekasu for her face. Sakekasu is leftover solids from the process of Sake production. Sakekasu or sake in general is known for its numerous benefits such as anti-ageing. It is an excellent product for our hair.

## Sake: A different form of fermented rice

Sake is a type of rice wine produced in Japan and has been a crucial part of its culture for as long as hundreds of years. It is an alcoholic beverage brewed by microbes called Koji and fermented by yeast. Sake is mainly composed of water, ethanol, glycerol, organic acids, amino acids and ethyl D-glucoside. This compound also corresponds to sake's distinct taste.

Sake is great for hair and Japanese people use it to get softer skin and hair. Ethyl D glycoside in sake has anti-ageing benefits and also restores the natural skin barrier and prevents damage associated with UV radiation. Ferulic acid, naturally present in rice, is a potent antioxidant and anti-inflammatory agent. Adenosine and its analogues are present in sake. The topical application of adenosine has proven to be effective in inducing hair growth for both males and females suffering from androgenic alopecia. Ethanol in sake has antimicrobial properties and will help in treating dandruff.

**Incorporating these Japanese practices may help you upgrade your hair game and achieve your hair goals. Here are some hair masks that can help you get healthy, strong and luscious hair.**

# Natural hair masks

## Sake-citron mask for dandruff

**Ingredients**

- Juice from 1 yuzu or lemon
- 1 tbsp honey
- 2 tbsp sake

Yuzu, also called Japanese citron, is a citrus fruit grown in east Asian countries such as China, Japan and Korea. It is abundant in flavonoids, carotenoids, Vitamin B complex, Vitamin C, tannins, anthocyanins, phenolic acids, etc. which makes it a strong antioxidant fruit. Yuzu has a strong antimicrobial activity similar to lemons and can be used to combat dandruff-causing bacteria and fungi. Honey is a natural humectant and provides moisture and shine to hair. It is also proven to be effective in treating and preventing dandruff and seborrheic dermatitis.

Sake is mainly composed of water, ethanol, glycerol, organic acids, amino acids and ethyl D-glucoside. Sake has anti-ageing, antimicrobial and antioxidant effects, and people in Japan use it to acquire softer skin and hair.

Mix everything well. Apply this mixture to dry or slightly damp hair (scalp and roots only). Keep it on for around 10-20 minutes then wash with a mild shampoo. Do this twice a week and continue it for 2-3 weeks to eliminate dandruff. You can see the difference within a single wash.

## Seaweed as a natural cleanser for oily hair

### Ingredients

- 1 tsp Funori powder
- 1 cup water

Seaweed is one of the most important ingredients in Japanese food. But apart from that, it also holds important cosmetic value. Shampoos became a norm in Japan only in the last century. Before that, people used natural remedies to cleanse their hair. Japanese people used to use seaweed powder as a natural shampoo as seaweed has a neutral pH of 6.5, has oceanic aromas and leaves the scalp sebum and dirt free without over-drying. Unlike Funori, shampoos are alkaline, disturb the natural balance of the scalp and over-dry it, which then causes excess sebum production in response. Red algae is rich in essential amino acids, omegas 3 and 6 fatty acids, iron, iodine, phosphorus and calcium, Vitamins B2 and B12 and beta carotene.

Funori is a red alga available as a mix of 3 types of seaweeds *fukuro-funori*, *ma-kombu*, and *mekabu*, and it is used in powder form. It might take a couple of weeks for your hair to get used to not shampooing. Your hair might feel oilier or drier during this period. The hair will normalize itself eventually. If completely ditching shampoo isn't possible for you, you can also mix seaweed powder with a small amount of mild sulfate-free shampoo.

Mix seaweed powder with water. Wash your hair with lukewarm water and apply the seaweed mixture to your hair and gently massage with your fingertips. Rinse it off with water after.

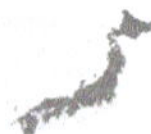

## Japanese hair oil for hair growth

**Ingredients**

- Camellia oil
- Sesame oil
- Walnut oil

Camellia oil is the most common hair oil used in Japan due to its numerous benefits. It is high in good fatty acids, vitamins and minerals. It contains twice as much Vitamin E as olive oil and also contains more monounsaturated fatty acids (almost 90%). It is also abundant in squalene and flavonoids. Triacylglycerols are the major components of walnuts including both mono and polyunsaturated fatty acids, especially omega-3 fatty acids. It is also rich in folates and other forms of Vitamins B, C, E and K. Iron and zinc, both essential for hair health, are also abundant. Due to their high phenolic and polyphenolic content, these are potent antioxidants.

Sesame oil is another popular oil in Japan and other east Asian countries. It is an excellent source of sulfur-containing amino acids, fatty acids, copper and calcium. Scientific studies have identified its hair growth-promoting potential as well.

Mix all oils and store the mixture in a glass bottle. Apply this oil before your shower, massage gently and keep it in for 2-4 hours. Rinse it off with a mild shampoo. You can apply a few drops of camellia oil after a shower on damp hair as well to make it more manageable.

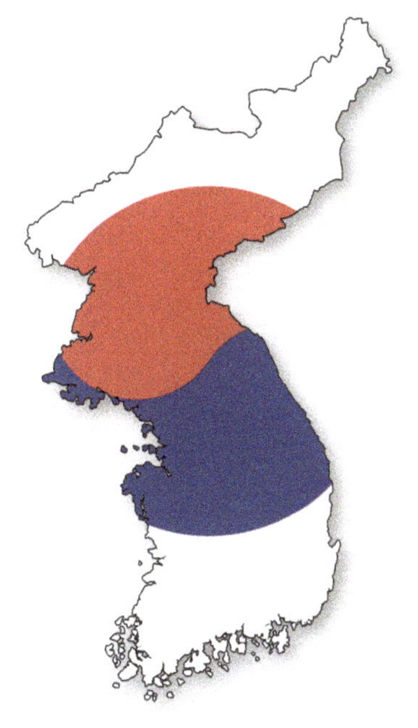

# KOREA

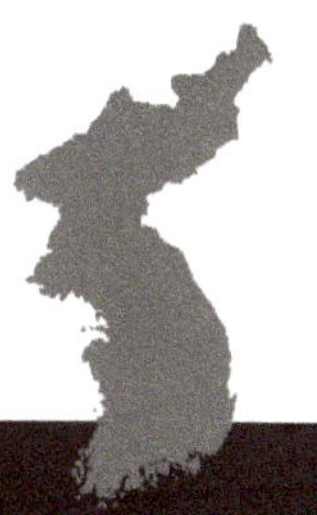

# Introduction

South Korea is well known for its beauty secrets that have helped them achieve beautiful glowing skin and soft, dark and luscious hair. They are very considerate of first impressions and put great effort into maintaining their skin and hair health. According to South Koreans, the scalp's health is as important as their skin and they believe that it reflects hair quality. They have found a balance between natural remedies and commercial products, by combining oil treatments and other natural ingredients with products like hair essences, masks and serums in their regimen to get maximum benefit.

## Korean hair routine: More meticulous than skincare

We all know about Korean skincare and the numerous steps involved in it. It is a very elaborate yet effective routine and transforms the skin. Korean hair care, on the other hand, is often overlooked. It is a multi-step routine with each step important and adding to the benefits. Here are all the steps to do a Korean regimen at home.

### 1- Scalp scaler

Once a week, Koreans use a scalp scaler to exfoliate and remove dead skin, sebum and product buildup. It is similar to face peels as it is made of salicylic acid. It does not lather and is applied before shampoo.

### 2- Shampoo

They prefer a mild shampoo that also balances the scalp's ph.

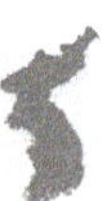

### 3- Conditioner

Conditioner is followed by shampoo as usual to moisturize the hair.

### 4- Scalp massage

Scalp massagers with gentle bristles are available all over Korea. These improve blood circulation without causing breakage. Use this once the hair completely dries off as wet hair is very fragile.

### 5-Hair mask

Koreans love hydrating masks. Ingredients such as seaweed, rice, banana, avocado, coconut, etc., are commonly used. A Korean rapper, CL, also advocates its benefits, saying she uses a hair mask treatment at least once a week.

### 6-Toners

We have all heard of facial toners, but most of us would not know about scalp and hair toners. These toners help in soothing inflammation and itchiness, plus assist with combating dandruff. Hydrating toners can relieve dry and flaky scalp.

### 7- Essences and serums

The last step of the routine is to apply a serum or essence. Essences are a very commonly used product in South Korea and are essentially lightweight versions of serums. They moisturize the hair without making it greasy. These serums are also available for the scalp and are used to enhance hair growth.

### Healthy diet = Healthy hair

It is a world-known fact that no routine, no remedy can match diet. A balanced healthy diet is the first step in achieving hair and skin goals

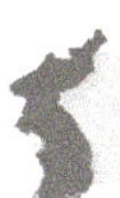



and without it, every effort is futile. Kimchi, a staple fermented food in Korea, is rich in probiotics, vitamins and antioxidants. One study even provides evidence that probiotics in kimchi can help improve androgenic alopecia. Koreans also have a high intake of seafood, which is rich in omega-3 fatty acids and lean protein.

## Koreans love their hair rinses

Hair rinses are pretty popular throughout the world, and Korea is no exception. Rice water is extremely common over there and has been used for centuries to promote hair growth. Rice is also the main ingredient in many of their haircare products. Other than that, vinegar rinses are also used to remove dandruff and product buildup. You can make your own apple cider vinegar rinse by mixing 1 part ACV with 2 parts water. Apply after shampooing, leave it on for 5 minutes and rinse it with water.

## Argan oil

Argan oil, although not native to Korea, has been a part of Korean hair care for a long time. A South Korean singer, Kim Yu-jin, also called Uee, from the kpop group Afterschool, says that she applies Moroccan argan oil every day to protect her hair from damage caused by constant styling and dyeing.

## A quick fix to tame frizzy hair

Korean actress **Yoon Eun Hye** shared her secret of an instant fix for a bad hair day. She recommends using 2-3 drops mixed with water to tame frizz and split ends. Another solution is to use facial hydrating mists or moisturizers on hair to reduce dryness and frizz, recommended by a famous model named Kim Irene.

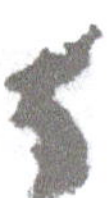

# Natural hair masks

## Coffee shampoo for hair growth and dandruff

**Ingredients**

- 1 glass of warm water
- 2-3 tbsp of coffee
- ½ tsp salt
- 3-4 tbsp of baby shampoo
- 1 tsp coconut oil
- 1 tsp honey

Coffee is rich in antioxidants and caffeine, which is a stimulant and increases blood flow to the scalp. Various studies have been conducted to check its effect on patients suffering from hair loss. Many studies have confirmed that caffeine can inhibit testosterone-induced growth inhibition that occurs in male and female pattern baldness. It is shown to increase hair thickness and density. Coffee can also help in temporary coverage of grey hair and control dandruff. Salt helps clean hair by removing oil and dirt. Coconut oil and honey will moisturize the hair, providing it with nutrients that will strengthen the hair and give a natural shine to the strands.

Mix everything thoroughly. Apply on dry hair, and massage gently so that it lathers and spreads across the entire scalp. Leave it on for 15 minutes. Wash with warm water and use a conditioner after. This shampoo is great for people with oily scalp type. You can also skip the coconut oil if you want more volume.

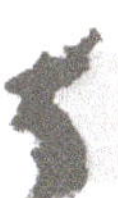



## Conditioning rice hair mask for dry and damaged hair

**Ingredients**

- ¼ cup rice
- 1 cup water
- 2 tbsp argan oil
- 3 drops lavender essential oil

Rice water is one of the most common haircare remedies that has been used for many years in the countries of Japan, China and Korea due to its immense benefits. Here's a rice recipe that you can say is an upgrade from rice water and will help you get super soft hair. Inositol, a type of Vitamin B present in rice, can penetrate and repair the hair. Rice is also rich in peptides that can strengthen hair and will prevent hair breakage. Rice has anti-inflammatory and moisturizing properties due to the phenolic compounds present such as squalene, betaine and tricin. Argan oil is also rich in peptides and will deeply moisturize the hair. The lavender essential oil will leave your hair smelling lovely.

Add the rice and water to a pot, cover and cook it well. The rice should be mushy and moist, not dry. Take 2 tbsp of that mixture, and add in the argan oil and lavender essential oil. Blend it with the help of a food processor. The consistency should be smooth and thick, similar to normal conditioners. Section your hair and apply this to the entire hair shaft, roots to ends and leave it for 1-2 hours. Cover it with a shower cap and wash it off with warm water.

This mask is ideal for extremely dry hair that results in tangling and breakage. It will soften the hair and provide shine. The hair will be much more manageable even after a single use.

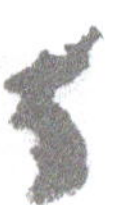

## A DIY Korean hair essence/gel for soft and glossy hair

**Ingredients**

- 8 drops milk thistle essential oil
- 8 drops Korean red ginseng/ Panax ginseng essential oil
- Aloe vera gel
- 1 Vitamin E capsule OR 1 tsp Vitamin E oil

Silymarin milk thistle is rich in flavonoids such as a flavonolignan called Silibinin, which is its major active component. These flavonoids are potent antioxidants, and therefore, the plant has been used in Korean folk medicine for a very long time. It also can reduce inflammation. The hair growth-promoting benefits of ginseng had previously been mentioned as well in the section on China. In a study conducted in South Korea, milk thistle was proven to improve the texture of damaged hair. Red ginseng contains ginsenosides and other active substances that are anti-inflammatory, antioxidant and also anti-DHT, which is the culprit of androgenetic alopecia. It also upregulates keratin-producing cells in the hair matrix. Aloe vera has moisturizing properties and will serve as a medium for the application and absorption of these oils in the hair. Vitamin E is a strong antioxidant and deeply moisturizes and nourishes the hair shaft.

Take organic aloe vera gel and mix the essential oils and the Vitamin E capsule in it. Do not use fresh aloe vera gel. Stir them thoroughly to emulsify everything together. It will turn white and creamy from transparent and gel-like. Keep mixing till the colour is changed to white completely. You can store this in the refrigerator for a week. For application, take a little bit in your fingertips and run through the ends of your hair to provide shine and tame frizz.

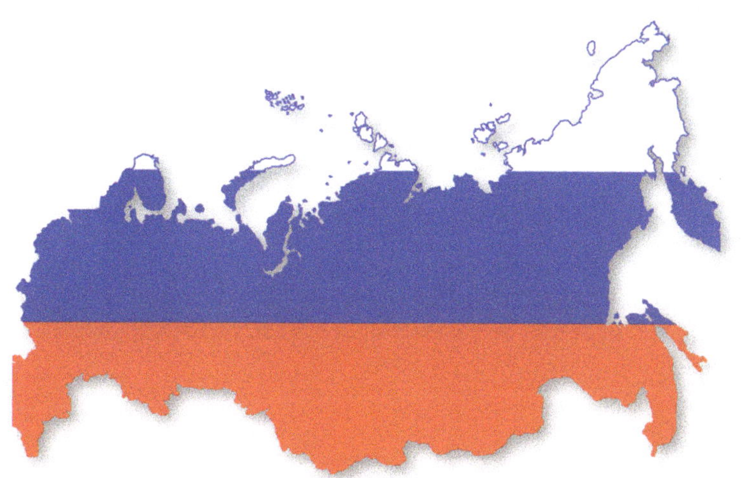

# Russia

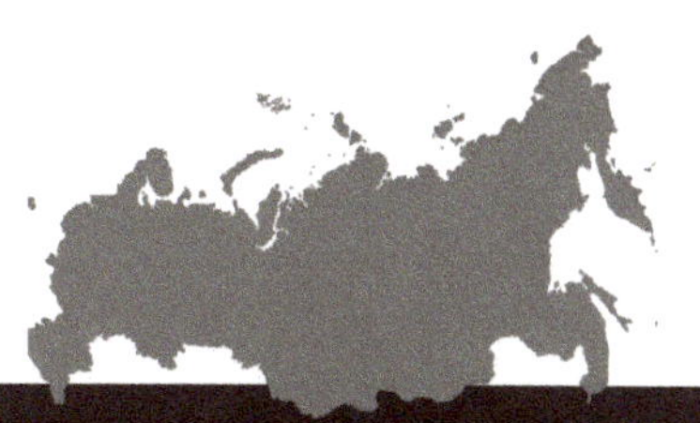

# Introduction

Hair has been a symbol of beauty and health for centuries and healthy hair can drastically affect your appearance. Russians are famous for their beautiful skin and long hair. Diving into the use of natural products and their other haircare secrets can help us achieve our hair goals. Russian haircare is all about maintaining scalp health and balancing its pH. The hair can only be healthy if the scalp is. They use various hair tonics, and herbal and natural masks to grow hair and get rid of hair problems such as dandruff, hair fall, etc.

## Herbal remedies

Russia is the place for getting herbs as they are readily available and very cheap. Herbs such as stinging nettle, clover, hibiscus, plantain, etc., are all great for hair growth and can be easily found there. Some people even recommend directly rubbing their juice on the scalp. However, recipes for effective natural hair masks have been given below that can help you achieve your Russian hair fantasy.

## Alcohol is where it's at

Alcohol is very popular in Russia considering their climate—but not just for drinking. It is also used to make hair tonics to make your hair grow. Vodka and cayenne tonic is an extremely popular one that has been used for hundreds of years in Russia. The detailed recipe for this tonic is mentioned below. An accomplished actress, writer and director, **Renata Litvinova**, has shared her favourite alcohol, saying she rubs burr oil mixed with egg yolks and cognac on her hair.

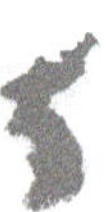

## Back to the basics

Identifying your hair type and your hair's needs can help you choose relevant products. Russians love to use mild shampoos plus weekly keratin or other hydrating masks to maintain their hair health. You can also use natural hair masks along with these to further increase the benefits. Regular application of oils is also a common practice in Russia to fortify the hair. Also, take enough sun and supplements of biotin and omega 3 for strong, thick and radiant hair.

## Take some steam

Russia used to have very popular steaming places similar to saunas called "Banyas." These Banyas used to be available for hygiene purposes but are still quite popular in Russia today. Steam can help open hair cuticles and allow better product penetration. Steaming is especially beneficial for people with low porosity hair, as the hair usually struggles to take up moisture; steam can help with that and will also improve blood circulation.

# Natural hair masks

## Mustard hair growth mask:

Ingredients

- 1 tbsp mustard powder
- 2 tbsp sugar
- 2 tbsp mayonnaise
- 2 tbsp olive oil

Mustard is rich in Vitamins A and E and omega-3 fatty acids; it will nourish the hair roots, making them healthier and stronger. Mayonnaise is essentially eggs and oil. It is rich in proteins, fatty acids and vitamins. It is a great treatment to get softer, healthier and shinier hair. This mask is ideal for weak, brittle hair that refuses to grow at all. It will provide hydration, strength and elasticity to the hair and you will notice a significant increase in hair growth.

Mix everything. If the mixture is too thick, you can add a dash of water to loosen it. Consistency should be similar to mayo or sour cream, i.e., not too runny but not too thick either. Apply it for 15-30 minutes and rinse it off. Initially, add 1 tbsp of sugar to the mask and gradually increase it to 2 after a few weeks. Sugar makes the mustard stronger/more potent, so using a high amount of sugar at first may irritate. While rinsing the mask, make sure to avoid contact with the face, especially the eyes. Use this once a week.

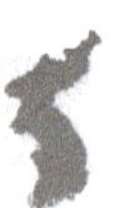

## Cayenne-ACV rinse for oily hair

**Ingredients**

- ½ tsp cayenne pepper powder (without any additives)
- 2-3 tbsp apple cider vinegar
- 1 cup warm water

Cayenne pepper may sound like a very unusual ingredient to be putting on our hair, but that is not the case in Russia. Cayenne-infused vodka is one of the most common haircare recipes used in Russia. Cayenne peppers contain a compound called Capsaicin; the same compound that causes the burning sensation when you eat any spicy food. Capsaicin increases blood circulation on the scalp and will help in hair growth. Apple cider vinegar is a great clarifying agent and will get rid of any buildup, grease and debris on the scalp.

Mix cayenne pepper with apple cider vinegar in warm water. Rinse your hair with this mixture after shampooing and keep it for 5-10 minutes. Wash it off with water. Do these 3-4 times a week to ensure proper scalp clarification and prevention of any buildup.

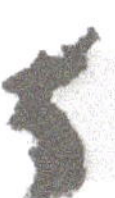



## Cayenne-Vodka hair tonic: A Russian hair secret

### Ingredients

- 1 cup fresh cayenne pepper
- 2 cups vodka (80%)

A traditional haircare recipe that is very common among babushkas is cayenne-infused vodka. It has been used for many centuries to enhance hair growth, improve the quality of the locks and balance the scalp's pH.

The two important components of cayenne are isoflavone and capsaicin. Research studies have identified that isoflavone and capsaicin administration on the scalp promotes the production of insulin-like growth factor 1, increasing hair growth. Cayenne is rich in carotenoids; a pigment responsible for its vibrant colour and possesses anti-inflammatory and antioxidant properties. Capsaicin also helps in blood stimulation on the scalp. It has been indicated by scientific evidence that cayenne has anagen stimulation, anti-baldness and hair growth-promoting properties.

Fill an airtight glass jar with vodka, add the peppers to it and store for a week in a dark place. Strain the mixture and you can now use this tonic on your hair. Wet your hair before using, leave it on for half an hour and rinse it off. Use it no more than once a week.

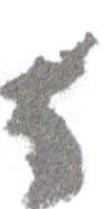

## Nicotinic Acid for fast hair growth

Ingredients

- 1 tbsp niacin powder / 2 niacin capsules / 1 niacin ampoule

Nicotinic acid—also called niacin, Vitamin PP, or B3—is a water-soluble vitamin. It is essential for the external and internal health of our body. Niacin increases protein (keratin) synthesis in hair, strengthening it and reducing hair loss. It has anti-inflammatory and antioxidant properties and can soothe an irritated scalp. It can also help with dandruff and greasy hair; there is scientific evidence about niacinamide, a milder form of niacin, reducing sebum production in the skin. In Russia, it is usually available in ampoule form and people rub these directly on their scalp to get long hair. Although, you should take breaks after 3-4 weeks of application as too much usage may cause more harm than good.

The texture is light and non-greasy and therefore application will be seamless. Niacin is commonly available as a powder at any local pharmacy. You can also get it in capsule form and take the powder out. Dissolve this in a little bit of water to make a thin watery mixture and apply it on the scalp to induce overall hair growth. You can also apply it only to the thinning spots to induce hair regrowth.

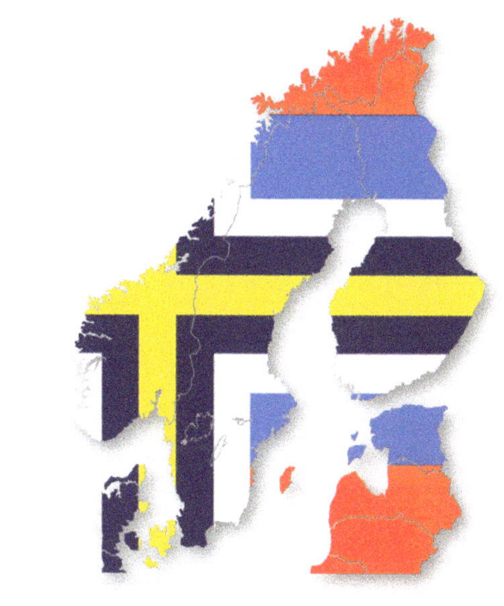

# Scandinavia

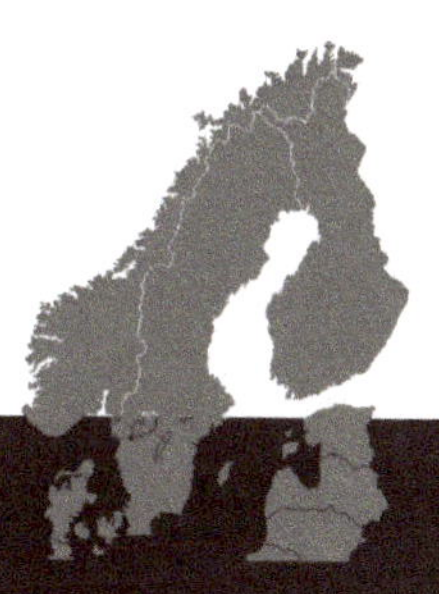

# Introduction

Striking blonde hair and bright blue eyes are the look of Nordic women, i.e., residing in the countries of Sweden, Norway, Iceland, Finland, Denmark, etc. The women there believe in a more holistic approach to beauty. This means that emphasis on whole body health is given to ensure hair and skin health as well. Eating well, supplements, exercising and reducing stress are all things they do along with the natural targeted treatments.

## Glacier water

We are 70% water, and therefore, water quality has a drastic effect on our health. Scandinavian regions have a very cold climate with glaciers and mountains found almost everywhere. This water is free of harmful chemicals and minerals, unlike the ones that we usually get in our homes. Hard water is one of the most common causes of hair fall and makes your hair appear frizzy and rough. Using glacier water makes your hair soft and manageable and drinking it also has numerous health benefits.

## Clean is always better

Scandinavian people love natural organic products and avoid harsh chemicals such as sulfates, parabens and silicones. These chemicals make the hair extremely dry, weak and dull. They also eat organic, unprocessed food, especially fish and other types of seafood. Fish is rich in omega-3 fatty acids, which are excellent for boosting hair growth and making you thicker and fuller. Cloudberries are a quite popular fruit with numerous health benefits and are also a part of many haircare formulations there, such as shampoos and

conditioners. Shark liver oil is a popular supplement in Scandinavia and is an excellent source of squalene, plus it helps in moisture retention.

## Sauna

Saunas are pretty popular in Norwegian regions and rightfully so. Steam in saunas helps in the rejuvenation of skin and hair, improves blood circulation and also triggers collagen and keratin synthesis in the cells. It also assists in reducing stress, which we all know is not good for us and our hair.

## Balance is key

As mentioned before, Scandinavians are all about a holistic approach and achieving balance. Concepts like "hygge", which means to create a warm and comfortable environment, and "lagom", corresponding to doing everything in a balanced way, are key to their health. They do not fuss about being perfect and consider their physical, mental and social health altogether, tending to each equally.

## It's not that complicated

Talented and famous Swedish singer **Lykke Li** has shared her love for natural products, especially oils, in an interview. She likes to keep a minimalistic routine, loves to mix oils like jojoba, almond and grapeseed in her beauty routine and uses coconut oil on her hair often.

# Natural hair masks

## Egg-banana deep conditioning treatment

**Ingredients**

- 2 egg yolks
- 2 bananas
- 2 tsp honey
- 2 tbsp olive oil
- 6 tbsp of hair conditioner (depends on your hair length)

Weak brittle hair is one of the most frustrating hair problems to encounter. Weak hair can appear frizzy and dull, and it can also cause a lot of breakages. If your hair is very dry, thinning and breaking off, you are in dire need of a deep conditioning/protein treatment. The egg is a source of complete protein, i.e., it has all the essential amino acids that the body can not produce itself. The yolk is more concentrated in nutrients than egg whites and will provide you with all the care you need. Bananas are a rich source of potassium, magnesium and Vitamins A, C, B6 and B12. The bananas along with honey will provide shine and moisture to your hair and will keep dandruff at bay due to their hygroscopic and antimicrobial properties.

Blend the yolks, banana, honey and olive oil. Mix it in with the hair conditioner and apply from the mid to the end sections of the hair. Do not apply to roots or scalp. Leave it on for 30 minutes and rinse it with water. Shampoo before applying the mask so that the hair is clean for a deep conditioning treatment. Your hair will visibly be more manageable, soft and shiny upon using this mask just once.

## Ginger-yoghurt mask for dandruff and itchy scalp

**Ingredients**

- 4 tbsp ginger juice
- 2 tbsp lemon juice
- ¼ cup yoghurt

Ginger has anti-inflammatory, antioxidant and antimicrobial properties and can help calm the inflamed and itchy scalp. Along with that, it can be beneficial in stimulating blood circulation in the scalp and preventing hair fall. Lemon juice is one of the most effective natural ingredients to combat dandruff due to its strong antibacterial and antifungal activity. Yoghurt is full of probiotics, healthy fats, amino acids, vitamins like B2 and B12, and minerals such as calcium, magnesium and zinc. It will help provide nourishment to the scalp, which is essential to maintaining healthy hair.

Extract juice of around a 2-inch piece of ginger or enough to make 3-4 tbsp of juice. Add to yoghurt and lemon juice and mix it well till smooth. Apply this mask for 1 hour, before shampooing, and then rinse it off. Repeat it once a week.

## Cinnamon for hair loss and regrowth

### Ingredients

- 2 tbsp cinnamon powder
- 4 tbsp coconut oil (Any oil of your choice)

Cinnamon might sound weird to be putting on our hair, but it is an excellent remedy for combating hair loss and baldness. A scientific study showed cinnamon oil to be as effective as minoxidil, which is the gold standard for stimulating new hair growth. It is rich in Vitamin A, iron and antioxidants and will help in improving blood circulation on your scalp and reducing hair fall.

Slightly warm up the oil and mix the cinnamon in it. Apply it to the scalp and toots and massage gently while applying. Let this sit for around 30-40 minutes and wash it off. Do not repeat this more than twice a week.

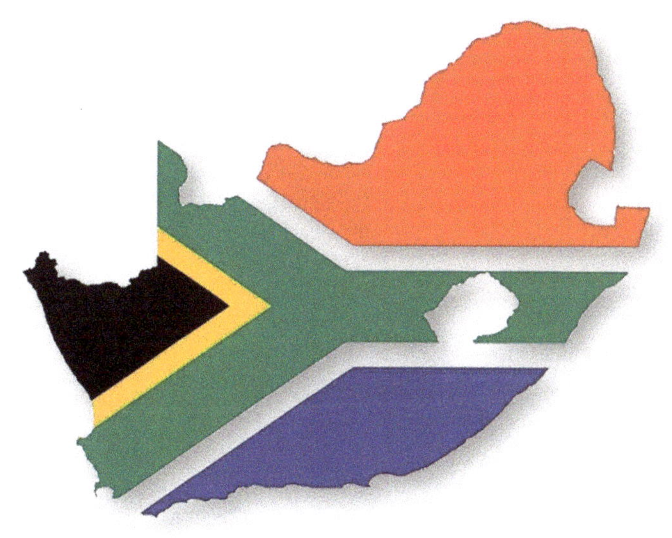

# South Africa

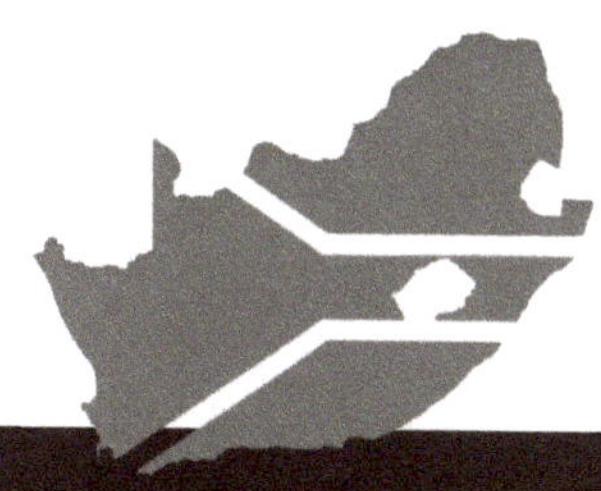

# Introduction

South Africans are famous for their signature thick, beautiful and dark curls. Ever wondered how they managed to achieve such strong, healthy and luscious hair? The answer to that is that African countries are very much keen on using natural ingredients and the grandmas have been using natural remedies to protect and nourish their hair for generations. These remedies are prevalent to this day. They love to hydrate their hair and define their curls, and for that, they regularly use deep conditioning treatments.

## African black soap

This is an all-natural soap, with antibacterial and antifungal properties. These soaps are traditionally black or dark brown and are used for skin and hair in Africa. It is unscented, has moisturizing properties and is made of ingredients like shea butter, honey and palm oil with the ash of burnt plantain skin or cocoa pod. Many brands of soap are available worldwide, and you can use it in place of shampoo to get rid of dandruff due to its antimicrobial properties.

## Butters and ghee

Africans love to use deeply moisturizing treatments due to their thick hair texture. Ghee, which is a common African and east Asian ingredient, is made by clarifying butter and is usually liquid at room temperature. Ghee is full of saturated fats and nutrients that help in strengthening and hydrating the hair. Aside from ghee, various kinds of butter such as shea butter and avocado butter are also very commonly used along with oils like argan and marula oil. Some African oil recipes are also mentioned below. South African actress and model Pearl Thusi also gave the tip of using organic oils and butter on damp hair. She loves jojoba oil, avocado oil and shea butter.

## Rooibos tea

South Africans love to drink rooibos tea, also called red tea. It is a non-caffeinated drink and is full of antioxidants and is a rich source of copper and fluoride. It is made by fermenting leaves of a species called *Aspalathus linearis*. It's usually drunk like black tea, with milk and sugar. The tea also has hair growth-promoting effects and is used as a hair rinse by Southern African women.

## Wash your hair less

Now, this depends on your hair type, of course, but Africans wash their hair very infrequently. They usually braid, thread their hair, or get dreadlocks. Due to their hair's texture, hair washing is a long process, and it is also not healthy for the hair to be washed every day. However, not washing enough can also lead to scalp buildup and clogged pores, which is not healthy for the hair either. **Nomzamo Mbatha**, a South African actress, shared in an interview how she prefers washing her hair once a week. Moisturizing is key, so make sure to always condition after washing your hair and use a deep conditioning mask once a week.

# Natural hair masks

## Hot-oil treatment for dandruff and hair growth

**Ingredients**

- 1 tsp coconut oil
- 1 tsp jojoba oil
- 1 tsp Jamaican black castor oil
- 10 drops tea tree oil

Do you always struggle with a frizzy dry mess despite putting countless conditioners and serums on your hair? Does your hair easily get tangled and is hard to manage? Chances are that you might have low porosity hair, i.e., your hair can't absorb moisture well. Coconut, jojoba and Jamaican black castor oils are a few of the most common and effective oils used in South Africa. These oils have amino acids, vitamins and fatty acids, all of which are essential for healthy hair. These moisturize the hair along with strengthening and aiding in hair growth. Warming up oils allows greater penetration into the hair shaft ensuring absorption and long-term moisture retention. Tea tree oil has anti-bacterial and anti-fungal properties and will get rid of that stubborn dandruff in no time!

Prepare a double boiler, i.e., boil water in a pot and place an empty bowl above it. Make sure the bowl does not directly touch the water. This method ensures that the oils are not overheated. Heat all the oils together except tea tree oil. Add tea tree oil once the oils are warmed up. Apply it to the scalp and roots and massage gently for 5 minutes. You can also steam your hair for additional benefits by better penetration of the oils into the scalp. Rinse with shampoo after 2-4 hours. You can repeat this once a week.

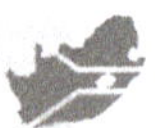

## Henna- A natural hair dye and conditioner

**Ingredients**

- 1 cup henna powder
- 3 tbsp lemon juice
- Water

Henna hair dye is a natural red/orange dye made by grinding henna leaves. Henna is a plant that holds great ethnobotanical relevance. Originating from the north of Africa and the Middle East, it has been widely used in various countries of Africa and Asia. Traditionally, it has been used to decorate hands and feet with artistic designs, usually for special occasions such as weddings, festivals, etc. Henna is rich in phytochemicals including lawsone, a naphthoquinone that gives its leaves the colouring properties. It is rich in antioxidants and has antimicrobial properties that your hair will benefit from.

Grind dried henna leaves or you can use henna powder and add lemon juice and water to make a smooth thick paste. Let it sit overnight. Cover with a cling wrap. Adding lemon juice helps to intensify the colour. Leave it for 2 hours. Use petroleum jelly on your face, neck and ears while applying the mask to prevent staining. It will last about 4-6 weeks. If you are using henna powder, make sure your henna is free of additives and harmful chemicals as henna adulteration is very common. Although generally safe, do a patch test before applying to check for any allergic reactions.

Henna deposits copper pigments deep into the hair shaft, and therefore, it would be best to avoid it in case you are planning to go blonde in the future.

## Lightweight anti-frizz oil for oily hair type

- 2 tbsp marula oil
- 2 tbsp baobab oil
- 2 tbsp argan oil

Frizziness of hair is one of the most frustrating hair problems that everyone is familiar with. While dry hair is usually more prone to frizz and split ends, people with an oily scalp are not always spared. Deep oil treatments aren't ideal for this type of hair as they affect hair volume and make it appear limp. Lighter oils can help tame any frizz and flyaways, without them appearing greasy or weighing the hair down.

Marula, argan and baobab oil are all native to African countries and are their age-old secret for moisturizing skin and hair. These oils are lightweight, non-irritating, hydrating and have occlusive properties that prevent moisture loss. These oils are rich in fatty acids including oleic acid, palmitic acid and stearic acid. They are rich in antioxidants such as Vitamin E, β-sitosterol, tyrosol, vanillic acid, ferulic acid and syringic acid. Argan oil is rich in squalene, which provides shine to the hair. These oils will lightly coat the hair shaft, making it softer, silkier and shinier.

Mix all the oils and store them in a glass dropper bottle. Apply a few drops of this oil after a shower on slightly damp hair. It is an excellent leave-in serum that will not weigh your hair down and will keep frizz away.

# References


1. Adhirajan, N., Ravi Kumar, T., Shanmugasundaram, N., & Babu, M. (2003). In vivo and in vitro evaluation of hair growth potential of Hibiscus rosa-sinensis Linn. *Journal of ethnopharmacology*, *88*(2-3), 235–239. https://doi.org/10.1016/s0378-8741(03)00231-9

2. Al-Waili, N. S. (2001). Therapeutic and prophylactic effects of crude honey on chronic seborrheic dermatitis and dandruff. *European Journal of Medical Research*, *6*(7), 306-308.

3. Anilakumar, K. R., Pal, A., Khanum, F., & Bawa, A. S. (2010). Nutritional, medicinal and industrial uses of sesame (Sesamum indicum L.) seeds-an overview. *Agriculturae Conspectus Scientificus*, *75*(4), 159-168.

4. Anis, M., Ahmed, S., & Hasan, M. M. (2017). Algae as nutrition, medicine and cosmetic: The forgotten history, present status and future trends. *World Journal of Pharmacy and Pharmaceutical Sciences*, *6*(6), 1934-1959.

5. Arun, P. P. S., Vineetha, Y., Waheed, M., & Ravikanth, K. (2019). Quantification of the minimum amount of lemon juice and apple cider vinegar required for the growth inhibition of dandruff causing fungi Malassezia furfur. *Int. J. Sci. Res. in Biological Sciences*, *6*(2).

6. Aziz, E., Batool, R., Khan, M. U., Rauf, A., Akhtar, W., Heydari, M., ... & Shariati, M. A. (2020). An overview on red algae bioactive compounds and their pharmaceutical applications. *Journal of Complementary and Integrative Medicine*, *17*(4).

7. Barsagade, P. D., Patil, P., & Umekar, M. J. (2020). A formulation of face pack and hair products of rice water for the use of skin and hair problem. *World Journal of Pharmacy and Pharmaceutical Sciences*, *9*(4), 683-694.

8. Barve, Kalyani & Dighe, Apurva (2016). *[SpringerBriefs in Molecular Science] The Chemistry and Applications of Sustainable Natural Hair Products || Hair Conditioner., 10.1007/978-3-319-29419-3 (Chapter 4), 37–44.* doi:10.1007/978-3-319-29419-3_4

9. Bassino, E., Gasparri, F., & Munaron, L. (2020). Protective role of nutritional plants containing flavonoids in hair follicle disruption: A review. *International Journal of Molecular Sciences, 21*(2), 523. https://doi.org/10.3390/ijms21020523

10. Bogaki, T., Mitani, K., Oura, Y., & Ozeki, K. (2017). Effects of ethyl-α-d-glucoside on human dermal fibroblasts. *Bioscience, Biotechnology, and Biochemistry, 81*(9), 1706-1711.

11. Branch, S. (2013). Fenugreek (Trigonella foenum-graecum L.) as a valuable medicinal plant. *International Journal of Advanced Biological and Biomedical Research, 1*, 922-931.

12. Branch, S. (2013). Fenugreek (Trigonella foenum-graecum L.) as a valuable medicinal plant. *International Journal of Advanced Biological and Biomedical Research, 1*, 922-931.

13. Burlando, B., & Cornara, L. (2013). Honey in dermatology and skin care: A review. *Journal of Cosmetic Dermatology, 12*(4), 306-313.

14. Choi B. Y. (2018). Hair-growth potential of ginseng and its major metabolites: A review on its molecular mechanisms. *International Journal of molecular Sciences, 19*(9), 2703. https://doi.org/10.3390/ijms19092703

15. Dąbrowska, M., Maciejczyk, E., & Kalemba, D. (2019). Rose hip seed oil: Methods of extraction and chemical composition. *European Journal of Lipid Science and Technology, 121*(8), 1800440.

16. Dasaroju, S., & Gottumukkala, K. M. (2014). Current trends in the research of Emblica officinalis (Amla): A pharmacological perspective. *Int J Pharm Sci Rev Res, 24*(2), 150-159.

17. Davoodi, M., Karimooy, F. N., Budde, T., Ortega-Martinez, S., & Moradi-Kor, N. (2019). Beneficial effects of Japanese sake yeast

supplement on biochemical, antioxidant, and anti-inflammatory factors in streptozotocin-induced diabetic rats. *Diabetes, Metabolic Syndrome and Obesity: Targets and Therapy, 12,* 1667–1673. https://doi.org/10.2147/DMSO.S220181

18. De Paepe, K., Hachem, J. P., Vanpee, E., Roseeuw, D., & Rogiers, V. (2002). Effect of rice starch as a bath additive on the barrier function of healthy but SLS-damaged skin and skin of atopic patients. *Acta dermato-venereologica, 82*(3), 184–186. https://doi.org/10.1080/00015550260132460

19. Draelos, Z. D., Jacobson, E. L., Kim, H., Kim, M., & Jacobson, M. K. (2005). A pilot study evaluating the efficacy of topically applied niacin derivatives for treatment of female pattern alopecia. *Journal of Cosmetic Dermatology, 4*(4), 258-261.

20. Draelos, Z. D., Matsubara, A., & Smiles, K. (2006). The effect of 2% niacinamide on facial sebum production. *Journal of Cosmetic and Laser Therapy, 8*(2), 96–101.

21. El Abbassi, A., Khalid, N., Zbakh, H., & Ahmad, A. (2014). Physicochemical characteristics, nutritional properties, and health benefits of argan oil: A review. *Critical Reviews in Food Science and Nutrition, 54*(11), 1401-1414.

22. El-Baroty, G. S., Abd El-Baky, H. H., Farag, R. S., & Saleh, M. A. (2010). Characterization of antioxidant and antimicrobial compounds of cinnamon and ginger essential oils. *African Journal of Biochemistry Research, 4*(6), 167-174.

23. El-Baroty, G. S., Abd El-Baky, H. H., Farag, R. S., & Saleh, M. A. (2010). Characterization of antioxidant and antimicrobial compounds of cinnamon and ginger essential oils. *African Journal of Biochemistry Research, 4*(6), 167-174.

24. Gad, H. A., Roberts, A., Hamzi, S. H., Gad, H. A., Touiss, I., Altyar, A. E., ... & Ashour, M. L. (2021). Jojoba Oil: An updated comprehensive review on chemistry, pharmaceutical uses, and toxicity. *Polymers, 13*(11), 1711.

25. Gad, H. A., Roberts, A., Hamzi, S. H., Gad, H. A., Touiss, I., Altyar, A. E., ... & Ashour, M. L. (2021). Jojoba oil: An updated comprehensive review on chemistry, pharmaceutical uses, and toxicity. *Polymers, 13*(11), 1711.

26. Gitanjali, D., Prajakta, P., Swati, B., Kiran, E., & Rajendra, B. (2014). Antimalassezia activity of medicated antidandruff shampoo formulated with microwave dried garlic powder with improved allicin stability. *The Natural Products Journal, 4*(1), 23-32.

27. Grant, J. E., Redden, S. A., & Chamberlain, S. R. (2019). Milk thistle treatment of children and adults with trichotillomania: A double-blind, placebo-controlled, cross-over negative study. *Journal of Clinical Psychopharmacology, 39*(2), 129.

28. Gubitosa, J., Rizzi, V., Fini, P., & Cosma, P. (2019). Hair care cosmetics: From traditional shampoo to solid clay and herbal shampoo, a review. *Cosmetics, 6*(1), 13.

29. Guillaume, D., & Charrouf, Z. (2011). Argan oil and other argan products: Use in dermocosmetology. *European Journal of Lipid Science and Technology, 113*(4), 403-408.

30. Hadi, H., Syed Omar, S. S., & Awadh, A. I. (2016). Honey, a gift from nature to health and beauty: A review. *British Journal of Pharmacy, 1*(1), 46-54

31. Harada, N.; Okajima, K. (2009). Effects of capsaicin and isoflavone on blood pressure and serum levels of insulin-like growth factor-I in normotensive and hypertensive volunteers with alopecia. *Biosci. Biotechnol. Biochem.* 2009, *73*, 1456–1459.

32. Hashizume, K., Ito, T., Shirato, K., Amano, N., Tokiwano, T., Ohno, T., ... & Okuda, M. (2020). Factors affecting levels of ferulic acid, ethyl ferulate and taste-active pyroglutamyl peptides in sake. *Journal of Bioscience and Bioengineering, 129*(3), 322-326.

33. Huh, S., Lee, J., Jung, E., Kim, S. C., Kang, J. I., Lee, J., ... & Park, D. (2009). A cell-based system for screening hair growth-promoting agents. *Archives of Dermatological Research, 301*(5), 381-385.

34. Inamasu, S., Ikuyama, R., Fujisaki, Y., & Sugimoto, K. I. (2010). Abstracts: The effect of rinse water obtained from the washing of rice (YU-SU-RU) as a hair treatment. *International Journal of Cosmetic Science, 32*(5), 392-393.

35. Indriana, L., Pangkahila, W., & Aman, I. G. M. (2018). Topical application of cinnamon (cinnamomum burmanii) essential oil has the same effectiveness as minoxidil in increasing hair length and diameter size of hair follicles in male white Wistar rats (rattus norvegicus). *IJAAM (Indonesian Journal of Anti-Aging Medicine), 2*(1), 13-16.

36. Jaafar, R. (2014). The effectiveness of coconut oil mixed with herbs to promote hair growth. International Journal of Ethics in Engineering & Management Education, 1(3), 27-30.

37. Jameel, M., & Ahmad, A. (2016). In vitro antibacterial, antifungal and GC-MS analysis of seeds of Mustard Brown. *Int j pharm Chem, 6*(4), 107-15.

38. Jang, S. H., Kim, M. J., Wee, J. H., Kim, J. T., & Choi, W. H. (2018). Effects of amla (Phyllanthus embilica L.) extract on hair growth promoting. *Korean Society for Biotechnology and Bioengineering Journal, 33*(4), 299-305.

39. Jolayemi, A. T., & Ojewole, J. A. O. (2013). Comparative anti-inflammatory properties of Capsaicin and ethylaAcetate extract of Capsicum frutescens linn [Solanaceae] in rats. *African Health Sciences, 13*(2), 357-361.

40. Kim, J. S., & Jeon, Y. H. (2021). Effects of milk thistle oil on chemically damaged hair improvement. *Journal of the Korean Applied Science and Technology, 38*(2), 434-440.

41. Kim, K. S. (2014). Research trends relevant with hair growth promotion and scalp condition improvement by applying natural extracts. *Kor J Aesthet Cosmetol, 12*(1), 17-24.

42. Kim, S. H., Jeong, K. S., Ryu, S. Y., & Kim, T. H. (1998). Panax ginseng prevents apoptosis in hair follicles and accelerates recovery of hair medullary cells in irradiated mice. *In vivo (Athens, Greece), 12*(2), 219-222.

43. Komane, B., Vermaak, I., Summers, B., & Viljoen, A. (2015). Safety and efficacy of Sclerocarya birrea (A. Rich.) Hochst (Marula) oil: A clinical perspective. *Journal of ethnopharmacology, 176*, 327-335.

44. Kong, M., & Kim, Y. (2010). Promotion effect of black sesame oil on hair growth in an alopecia model of C57BL/6 mice. *Journal of Biomedical Research, 11*(2), 103-116.

45. Kumar, K. S., Bhowmik, D., Duraivel, S., & Umadevi, M. (2012). Traditional and medicinal uses of banana. *Journal of Pharmacognosy and Phytochemistry, 1*(3), 51-63.

46. Levkovich, T., Poutahidis, T., Smillie, C., Varian, B. J., Ibrahim, Y. M., Lakritz, J. R., ... & Erdman, S. E. (2013). Probiotic bacteria induce a 'glow of health'. *PloS one, 8*(1), e53867.

47. Matsuda, H., Yamazaki, M., Asanuma, Y., & Kubo, M. (2003). Promotion of hair growth by ginseng radix on cultured mouse vibrissal hair follicles. *Phytotherapy Research, 17*(7), 797-800.

48. McKay, D. L., & Blumberg, J. B. (2006). A review of the bioactivity and potential health benefits of chamomile tea (Matricaria recutita L.). *Phytotherapy Research, 20*(7), 519-530.

49. McKay, D. L., & Blumberg, J. B. (2006). A review of the bioactivity and potential health benefits of chamomile tea (Matricaria recutita L.). *Phytotherapy Research, 20*(7), 519-530.

50. Mujoriya, R., & Bodla, R. B. (2011). A study on wheat grass and its nutritional value. *Food Science and Quality Management, 2*, 1-8.

51. Murata, K., Noguchi, K., Kondo, M., Onishi, M., Watanabe, N., Okamura, K., & Matsuda, H. (2013). Promotion of hair growth by Rosmarinus officinalis leaf extract. *Phytotherapy Research, 27*(2), 212-217.

52. Nahata, A., & Dixit, V. K. (2012). Ameliorative effects of stinging nettle (Urtica dioica) on testosterone-induced prostatic hyperplasia in rats. *Andrologia, 44*, 396-409.

53. Nakahara, M., Mishima, T., & Hayakawa, T. (2007). Effect of a sake concentrate on the epidermis of aged mice and confirmation of ethyl α-D-glucoside as its active component. *Bioscience, Biotechnology, and Biochemistry, 71*(2), 427-434.

54. Nakahara, M., Mishima, T., & Hayakawa, T. (2007). Effect of a sake concentrate on the epidermis of aged mice and confirmation of ethyl α-D-glucoside as its active component. *Bioscience, Biotechnology, and Biochemistry, 71*(2), 427-434.

55. Niharika, A., Aquicio, J. M., & Anand, A. (2010). Antifungal properties of neem (Azadirachta indica) leaves extract to treat hair dandruff. *E-ISRJ, 2*, 244-52.

56. Nile, S. H., & Park, S. W. (2014). Bioactive components and health-promoting properties of yuzu (Citrus ichangensis× C. reticulate). *Food Reviews International, 30*(2), 155-167.

57. Oh, G. N., & Son, S. W. (2012). Efficacy of korean red ginseng in the treatment of alopecia areata. *Journal of Ginseng Research, 36*(4), 391–395. https://doi.org/10.5142/jgr.2012.36.4.391

58. Oh, J. Y., Park, M. A., & Kim, Y. C. (2014). Peppermint oil promotes hair growth without toxic signs. *Toxicological Research, 30*(4), 297-304.

59. Oura, H., Iino, M., Nakazawa, Y., Tajima, M., Ideta, R., Nakaya, Y., Arase, S., & Kishimoto, J. (2008). Adenosine increases anagen hair growth and thick hairs in Japanese women with female pattern hair loss: a pilot, double-blind, randomized, placebo-controlled trial. *The Journal of Dermatology, 35*(12), 763–767. https://doi.org/10.1111/j.1346-8138.2008.00564.x

60. Panahi, Y., Taghizadeh, M., Marzony, E. T., & Sahebkar, A. (2015). Rosemary oil vs minoxidil 2% for the treatment of androgenetic alopecia: A randomized comparative trial. *Skinmed, 13*(1), 15-21.

61. Panahi, Y., Taghizadeh, M., Marzony, E. T., & Sahebkar, A. (2015). Rosemary oil vs minoxidil 2% for the treatment of androgenetic alopecia: a randomized comparative trial. *Skinmed, 13*(1), 15-21.

62. Parisi, O. I., Scrivano, L., Amone, F., Malivindi, R., Ruffo, M., Vattimo, A. F., ... & Puoci, F. (2018). Interconnected PolymerS TeChnology (IPSTiC): An effective approach for the modulation of 5α-reductase activity in hair loss conditions. *Journal of Functional Biomaterials, 9*(3), 44.

63. Park, G. H., Park, K. Y., Cho, H. I., Lee, S. M., Han, J. S., Won, C. H., ... & Lee, D. H. (2015). Red ginseng extract promotes the hair growth in cultured human hair follicles. *Journal of Medicinal Food, 18*(3), 354-362.

64. Park, G. H., Park, K. Y., Cho, H. I., Lee, S. M., Han, J. S., Won, C. H., Chang, S. E., Lee, M. W., Choi, J. H., Moon, K. C., Shin, H., Kang, Y. J., & Lee, D. H. (2015). Red ginseng extract promotes the hair growth in cultured human hair follicles. *Journal of Medicinal Food, 18*(3), 354–362. https://doi.org/10.1089/jmf.2013.3031

65. Paus R, Heinzelmann T, Schultz KD, et al. (1994). Hair growth induction by substance P. *Laboratory Investigation, 71*(1):134-140.

66. Paus, R., Heinzelmann, T., Schultz, K. D., Furkert, J., Fechner, K., & Czarnetzki, B. M. (1994). Hair growth induction by substance P. *Laboratory Investigation, 71*(1), 134-140.

67. Pekmezci, E., Dundar, C., & Turkoglu, M. (2018). Proprietary herbal extract downregulates the gene expression of IL-1α in HaCaT cells: Possible implications against nonscarring alopecia. *Medical Archives, 72*(2), 136.

68. Pieroni, A., Quave, C. L., Villanelli, M. L., Mangino, P., Sabbatini, G., Santini, L., ... & Tomasi, M. (2004). Ethnopharmacognostic survey on the natural ingredients used in folk cosmetics, cosmeceuticals and remedies for healing skin diseases in the inland Marches, Central-Eastern Italy. *Journal of Ethnopharmacology, 91*(2-3), 331-344.

69. Pieroni, A., Quave, C. L., Villanelli, M. L., Mangino, P., Sabbatini, G., Santini, L., ... & Tomasi, M. (2004). Ethnopharmacognostic survey on the natural ingredients used in folk cosmetics, cosmeceuticals and remedies for healing skin diseases in the inland Marches, Central-Eastern Italy. *Journal of Ethnopharmacology, 91*(2-3), 331-344.

70. Priya, K., Surabi, D., Sarath, R., & Mohandass, R. (2021). Isolation and characterization of active metabolites produced from probiotic isolates against dandruff causing malassezia furfur (MTCC: 1374T). *Journal of Microbiology, Biotechnology and Food Sciences, 10*(6), e3522-e3522.

71. Réhault-Godbert, S., Guyot, N., & Nys, Y. (2019). The golden egg: Nutritional value, bioactivities, and emerging benefits for human health. *Nutrients, 11*(3), 684.

72. Rele, A. S., & Mohile, R. B. (2003). Effect of mineral oil, sunflower oil, and coconut oil on prevention of hair damage. *Journal of Cosmetic Science, 54*(2), 175-192.

73. Rele, A. S., & Mohile, R. B. (2003). Effect of mineral oil, sunflower oil, and coconut oil on prevention of hair damage. *Journal of Cosmetic Science, 54*(2), 175–192.

74. Ryu, E. M., Seo, G. W., Kee, K. H., & Shin, H. J. (2013). Effect of ethanolic extract from wheat sprout on hair growth of C57BL/6 mouse. *Kor J Aesthet Cosmetol, 11*(6), 1051-1057.

75. Said, A. A. H., Otmani, I. S. E., Derfoufi, S., & Benmoussa, A. (2015). Highlights on nutritional and therapeutic value of stinging nettle (Urtica dioica). *International Journal of Pharmacy and Pharmaceutical Sciences, 7*(10), 8-14.

76. Sakthi, D. (2014). Effectiveness of fenugreek seed paste on dandruff among adolescent girls in selected women's hostel, Coimbatore. *International Journal of Nursing Education and Research, 2*(2), 147-150.

77. Salehi, B., Venditti, A., Sharifi-Rad, M., Kręgiel, D., Sharifi-Rad, J., Durazzo, A., Lucarini, M., Santini, A., Souto, E. B., Novellino, E., Antolak, H., Azzini, E., Setzer, W. N., & Martins, N. (2019). The therapeutic potential of apigenin. *International Journal of Molecular Sciences*, *20*(6), 1305.

78. Salehi, B., Venditti, A., Sharifi-Rad, M., Kręgiel, D., Sharifi-Rad, J., Durazzo, A., Lucarini, M., Santini, A., Souto, E. B., Novellino, E., Antolak, H., Azzini, E., Setzer, W. N., & Martins, N. (2019). The therapeutic potential of apigenin. *International Journal of Molecular Sciences*, *20*(6), 1305.

79. Satchell, A. C., Saurajen, A., Bell, C., & Barnetson, R. S. (2002). Treatment of dandruff with 5% tea tree oil shampoo. *Journal of the American Academy of Dermatology*, *47*(6), 852-855.

80. Satyal, P., Jones, T. H., Lopez, E. M., McFeeters, R. L., Ali, N. A., Mansi, I., Al-Kaf, A. G., & Setzer, W. N. (2017). Chemotypic characterization and biological activity of rosmarinus officinalis. *Foods (Basel, Switzerland)*, *6*(3), 20. https://doi.org/10.3390/foods6030020

81. Satyal, P., Jones, T. H., Lopez, E. M., McFeeters, R. L., Ali, N. A., Mansi, I., Al-Kaf, A. G., & Setzer, W. N. (2017). Chemotypic characterization and biological activity of rosmarinus officinalis. *Foods (Basel, Switzerland)*, *6*(3), 20. https://doi.org/10.3390/foods6030020

82. Semwal, R. B., Semwal, D. K., Combrinck, S., Cartwright-Jones, C., & Viljoen, A. (2014). Lawsonia inermis L.(henna): Ethnobotanical, phytochemical and pharmacological aspects. *Journal of Ethnopharmacology*, *155*(1), 80-103.

83. Semwal, R. B., Semwal, D. K., Combrinck, S., Cartwright-Jones, C., & Viljoen, A. (2014). Lawsonia inermis L.(henna): Ethnobotanical, phytochemical and pharmacological aspects. *Journal of Ethnopharmacology*, *155*(1), 80-103.

84. Shams-Ghahfarokhi, M., Shokoohamiri, M. R., Amirrajab, N., Moghadasi, B., Ghajari, A., Zeini, F., Sadeghi, G., & Razzaghi-Abyaneh, M. (2006). In vitro antifungal activities of Allium cepa, Allium sativum and ketoconazole against some pathogenic yeasts and dermatophytes. *Fitoterapia*, *77*(4), 321–323. https://doi.org/10.1016/j.fitote.2006.03.014

85. Sharma, L., Chandra, M., & Puneeta, A. (2020). Health benefits of lavender (Lavandula angustifolia). *International Journal of Physiology, Nutrition and Physical Education*, *4*(1), 1274-1277.

86. Singh, S., More, P. K., & Mohan, S. M. (2014). Curry leaves (Murraya koenigii Linn. Sprengal)-a mircale plant. *Indian Journal of Scientific Research*, *4*(1), 46-52.

87. Su, M. H., Shih, M. C., & Lin, K. H. (2014). Chemical composition of seed oils in native Taiwanese camellia species. *Food Chemistry*, *156*, 369-373.

88. Su, M. H., Shih, M. C., & Lin, K. H. (2014). Chemical composition of seed oils in native Taiwanese camellia species. *Food Chemistry*, *156*, 369-373.

89. Taha, N. A., & Al-wadaan, M. A. Significance and use of walnut, Juglans regia Linn: A review. *African Journal of Microbiology Research, 5*, 5796-5805. 10.5897/AJMR11.610.

90. Turnip, L., Sihotang, R. A., Turnip, K. N. T., & Arico, Z. (2018, September). The effect of coffee residu extract on hair growth. In *IOP Conference Series: Materials Science and Engineering* (Vol. 420, No. 1, p. 012079). IOP Publishing.

91. Umber, M., Sultana, R., Ijaz, T., & Aala, A. Leaf extract of Azadirachta indica (neem) as herbal cure of dandruff.

92. Vermaak, I., Kamatou, G. P. P., Komane-Mofokeng, B., Viljoen, A. M., & Beckett, K. (2011). African seed oils of commercial importance—Cosmetic applications. *South African Journal of Botany*, *77*(4), 920-933.

93. Völker, J. M., Koch, N., Becker, M., & Klenk, A. (2020). Caffeine and its pharmacological benefits in the management of androgenetic alopecia: A review. *Skin Pharmacology and Physiology, 33*(3), 153-169.

94. Wilson, E. A., & Demmig-Adams, B. (2007). Antioxidant, anti-inflammatory, and antimicrobial properties of garlic and onions. *Nutrition & Food Science, 37*(3), 178-183.

95. Zamil, D. H., Khan, R. M., Braun, T. L., & Nawas, Z. Y. (2022). Dermatological uses of rice products: trend or true?. *Journal of Cosmetic Dermatology,* 1-5.

96. Zargaran, A., Borhani-Haghighi, A., Faridi, P., Daneshamouz, S., Kordafshari, G., & Mohagheghzadeh, A. (2014). Potential effect and mechanism of action of topical chamomile (Matricaria chammomila L.) oil on migraine headache: A medical hypothesis. *Medical Hypotheses, 83*(5), 566-569.

## Photo Credits

Book Cover (James Montgomery, Cornell University PJ Mode Collection of Persuasive Cartography.) China, Italy, Korea, Russia, South Africa (www.pngwing.com); France (www.pngtree.com); India (www.pixabay.com); Japan (www.mappr.co); Scandinavia (www.commons.wikimedia.org).

www.ingramcontent.com/pod-product-compliance
Lightning Source LLC
Chambersburg PA
CBHW041300040426
42334CB00028BA/3095

* 9 7 8 0 6 4 6 8 7 4 8 1 4 *